Kendon J. Conrad, PhD
Cheryl I. Hultman, PhD
John S. Lyons, PhD

Treatment of the Chemically Dependent Homeless: Fourteen American Projects

SOME ADVANCE REVIEWS

"**T**his is a unique book that gets behind the summary data presented in most journal articles or book chapters, to tell the reader what it's "really like" to implement programs for homeless substance abusers and to research them. Because the scientific literature so often focuses on presenting the distilled "truth," we rarely get a chance to hear about the struggles of real people trying to get programs going, working with colleagues, government officials and fellow researchers in a very complex organizational arena. This volume presents, as well, an important perspective on the very real and very large problems providers encounter in their initial efforts to deliver high quality, often life-saving, services to homeless persons who suffer from substance abuse disorders. This book breathes new life into the phrase 'program implementation'."

Robert Rosenheck, MD
Director, VA Northeast Program
*   Evaluation Center*
Clinical Professor of Psychiatry
Yale University

"**T**he homeless who struggle to find sobriety and begin a stable recovery from alcoholism and drug abuse live in urban, suburban, and rural communities, and include the old and the young, women and men, drug addicts and alcoholics, and all races and ethnic groups. Many are challenged with serious mental illness. Services that promote recovery for homeless individuals, therefore, must recognize and respond to the diversity of the needs and characteristics they will encounter. *Treatment of the Chemically Dependent Homeless*, edited by Conrad, Hultman, and Lyons, describes 14 federally-funded projects designed to demonstrate and evaluate addiction treatment services for homeless men and women. Shelter providers, alcoholism and drug abuse counselors, case managers, and researchers will learn much. The volume documents program implementation and provides critical detail about program success and struggles. The heterogeneity of the target groups (e.g., public inebriates, women with children, veterans, Native Americans, and African Americans, dually-diagnosed) and multiplicity of interventions (e.g.,

case management, housing, residential care, day treatment) reflects the diversity of the need and means many can benefit from the experiences of the 14 projects. While all programs include case management components, the approaches vary and readers will learn from each. Denver is testing a case management dyad; in Washington D.C., they compare different case management models with mentally ill homeless alcoholics and addicts; St. Louis is working with women with children and providing family therapy; and Seattle's program for chronic public inebriates appears promising.

The implementation experiences are also valuable. Philadelphia's efforts to improve program retention among African American men using cocaine has much in common with the efforts in St. Louis to reduce dropouts among homeless mothers with children.

Political lessons are also apparent. New Orleans illustrates the deteriorative effects of turf issues and the need to influence political control. New Haven contrasts sharply and shows the value of compromise and collaboration.

Treatment of the Chemically Dependent Homeless complements earlier volume, *Treating Alcohol-ism and Drug Abuse Among the Homeless.* Together, they provide a complete overview of the 23 demonstration programs funded by the National Institute on Alcohol Abuse and Alcoholism in collaboration with the National Institute on Drug Abuse."

Dennis McCarty, PhD
Director
Bureau of Substance Abuse Services
Massachusetts Department
of Public Health

"**I** found *Treatment of the Chemically Dependent Homeless* to be particularly useful to both practitioners and researchers interested in exploring new and innovative ways to address the problems of the chemically dependent homeless. The book contains an introduction that provides the reader with a roadmap to better understand the forthcoming chapters. Each chapter presents an NIAA demonstration project. Most important is that many of the chapters provide feedback on problems or roadblocks that the demonstration project teams encountered as they went about developing and implementing the projects. The conclusion provides the reader with a comprehensive but concise summary of commonalities found in the chapters."

The Haworth Press, Inc.

John R. Belcher, PhD, LCSW
Associate Professor
School of Social Work
University of Maryland at Baltimore

Treatment of the Chemically Dependent Homeless: Fourteen American Projects

Treatment of the Chemically Dependent Homeless: Fourteen American Projects

Kendon J. Conrad, PhD
Cheryl I. Hultman
John S. Lyons
Editors

Treatment of the Chemically Dependent Homeless: Fourteen American Projects, edited by Kendon J. Conrad, Cheryl I. Hultman and John S. Lyons, was issued by The Haworth Press, Inc., under the title *Treatment of the Chemically Dependent Homeless: Theory and Implementation in Fourteen American Projects*, as a special issue of *Alcoholism Treatment Quarterly*, Volume 10, Numbers 3/4 1993, Thomas F. McGovern, Editor.

Harrington Park Press
An Imprint of
The Haworth Press, Inc.
New York · London

ISBN 1-56023-066-5

Published by

Harrington Park Press, 10 Alice Street, Binghamton, NY 13904-1580 USA

Harrington Park Press is an Imprint of the Haworth Press, Inc., 10 Alice Street, Binghamton, Ny 13904-1580 USA.

Treatment of the Chemically Dependent Homeless : Fourteen American Projects has also been published as *Alcoholism Treatment Quarterly*, Volume 10, Numbers 3/4 1993.

Library of Congress Cataloging-in-Publication Data

Treatment of the chemically dependent homeless : fourteen American projects / Kendon J. Conrad, Cheryl I. Hultman, John S. Lyons, editors.
    p. cm.
    Originally published : New York : Haworth Press, c1993.
    "Has also been published as Alcoholism treatment quarterly, volume 10, numbers 3/4, 1993"–T.p. verso.
    Includes bibliographical references and index.
    ISBN 1-56023-066-5
    1. Homeless persons–United States–Alcohol use. 2. Homeless persons–United States–Drug use. 3. Alcoholics–Rehabilitation–United States. 4. Narcotic addicts–Rehabilitation–United States. I. Conrad, Kendon J. II. Hultman, Cheryl I. III. Lyons, John (John S.)
[HV5140.T745 1995]
362.29'18'086942–dc20
                           95-4175
                           CIP

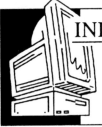

INDEXING & ABSTRACTING

Contributions to this publication are selectively indexed or abstracted in print, electronic, online, or CD-ROM version(s) of the reference tools and information services listed below. This list is current as of the copyright date of this publication. See the end of this section for additional notes.

- *Abstracts in Anthropology*, Baywood Publishing Company, 26 Austin Avenue, P.O. Box 337, Amityville, NY 11701

- *Abstracts of Research in Pastoral Care & Counseling*, Loyola College, 7135 Minstrel Way, Suite 101, Columbia, MD 21045

- *Addiction Abstracts*, National Addiction Centre, 4 Windsor Walk, London SE5 8AF, England

- *ALCONARC Database*, Swedish Council for Information on Alcohol and Other Drugs, Box 27302, S-102 54 Stockholm, Sweden

- *Cambridge Scientific Abstracts, Health & Safety Science Abstracts,* Cambridge Information Group, 7200 Wisconsin Avenue #601, Bethesda, MD 20814

- *Criminal Justice Abstracts*, Willow Tree Press, 15 Washington Street, 4th Floor, Newark, NJ 07102

- *Criminology, Penology and Police Science Abstracts*, Kugler Publications, P.O. Box 11188, 1001 GD Amsterdam, The Netherlands

- *Excerpta Medica/Electronic Publishing Division*, Elsevier Science Inc., Secondary Publishing Division, 655 Avenue of the Americas, New York, NY 10010

- *Index to Periodical Articles Related to Law*, University of Texas, 727 East 26th Street, Austin, TX 78705

- *Inventory of Marriage and Family Literature (online and hard copy)*, National Council on Family Relations, 3989 Central Avenue NE, Suite 550, Minneapolis, MN 55421

(continued)

- *Medication Use STudies (MUST) DATABASE*, The University of Mississippi, School of Pharmacy, University, MS 38677

- *Mental Health Abstracts (online through DIALOG)*, IFI/Plenum Data Company, 3202 Kirkwood Highway, Wilmington, DE 19808

- *NIAAA Alcohol and Alcohol Problems Science Database (ETOH)*, National Institute on Alcohol Abuse and Alcoholism, 1400 Eye Street NW, Suite 600, Washington, DC 20005

- *Psychological Abstracts (PsycINFO)*, American Psychological Association, P.O. Box 91600, Washington, DC 20090-1600

- *Referativnyi Zhurnal (Abstracts Journal of the Institute of Scientific Information of the Republic of Russia)*, The Institute of Scientific Information, Baltijskaja ul., 14, Moscow A-219, Republic of Russia

- *Social Planning/Policy & Development Abstracts (SOPODA)*, Sociological Abstracts, Inc., P.O. Box 22206, San Diego, CA 92192-0206

- *Social Work Research & Abstracts*, National Association of Social Workers, 750 First Street NW, 8th Floor, Washington, DC 20002

- *Sociological Abstracts (SA)*, Sociological Abstracts, Inc., P.O. Box 22206, San Diego, CA 92192-0206

- *SOMED (social medicine) Database*, Institute fur Dokumentation, Postfach 20 10 12, D-33548 Bielefeld, Germany

- *Studies on Women Abstracts*, Carfax Publishing Company, P.O. Box 25, Abingdon, Oxfordshire OX14 3UE, United Kingdom

- *The Brown University Digest of Addiction Theory and Application (DATA Newsletter)*, Project Cork Institute, Dartmouth Medical School, 14 South Main Street, Suite 2F, Hanover, NH 03755-2015

- *Violence and Abuse Abstracts: A Review of Current Literature on Interpersonal Violence (VAA)*, Sage Publications, Inc., 2455 Teller Road, Newbury Park, CA 91320

SPECIAL BIBLIOGRAPHIC NOTES

related to special journal issues (separates)
and indexing/abstracting

☐ indexing/abstracting services in this list will also cover material in any "separate" that is co-published simultaneously with Haworth's special thematic journal issue or DocuSerial. Indexing/abstracting usually covers material at the article/chapter level.

☐ monographic co-editions are intended for either non-subscribers or libraries which intend to purchase a second copy for their circulating collections.

☐ monographic co-editions are reported to all jobbers/wholesalers/approval plans. The source journal is listed as the "series" to assist the prevention of duplicate purchasing in the same manner utilized for books-in-series.

☐ to facilitate user/access services all indexing/abstracting services are encouraged to utilize the co-indexing entry note indicated at the bottom of the first page of each article/chapter/contribution.

☐ this is intended to assist a library user of any reference tool (whether print, electronic, online, or CD-ROM) to locate the monographic version if the library has purchased this version but not a subscription to the source journal.

☐ individual articles/chapters in any Haworth publication are also available through the Haworth Document Delivery Services (HDDS).

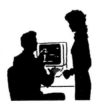

CONTENTS

POLITICS AND PROGRAMS: NEW ORLEANS, NEWARK, NEW HAVEN

SPECIAL POPULATIONS: ST. LOUIS, WASHINGTON, D.C.

TRANSITION TO INDEPENDENCE: BIRMINGHAM

CONCLUSION

ABOUT THE EDITORS

Kendon J. Conrad, PhD, is Research Associate Professor at the Center for Health Services and Policy Research of Northwestern University and Associate Director of the Midwest Health Services Research and Development Field Program of Hines VA Hospital. He has been principal, co-principal, or co-instigator on grants and contracts involving studies of the quality and effectiveness of health services. He has published research papers in major health and program evaluation journals and was principal investigator of the project described in this book.

Cheryl I. Hultman, PhD, is Research Assistant Professor at the Center for Health Services and Policy Research at Northwestern University and Research Health Scientist with the Midwest Health Services Research and Development Field Program at Hines VA Hospital. She has conducted research on the Department of Veterans Affairs Domiciliary Care Program for Homeless Veterans and the use of a psychiatric outreach team to reduce recidivism among patients with mental illness.

John S. Lyons, PhD, is Director of Research and Evaluation Services and Associate Professor of Psychiatry at Northwestern University Medical School. The author of more than 100 publications in the area of mental health services and policy research, Dr. Lyons is Faculty Director of Thresholds National Research and Training Center which studies community services for persons with psychiatric disabilities.

Introduction

Kendon J. Conrad, PhD
Cheryl I. Hultman, PhD
John S. Lyons, PhD

In 1990 the National Institute on Alcohol Abuse and Alcoholism (NIAAA) in cooperation with the National Institute on Drug Abuse funded fourteen research demonstration projects under Section 622 of the Stewart B. McKinney Homeless Assistance Act of 1988 (Public Law 100-628). The primary goal of these projects was to develop strategies or interventions to combat the dual problems of housing instability and substance abuse while simultaneously studying their effectiveness. In the following chapters, this NIAAA initiative and the fourteen projects funded under its auspices are described.

This book has two goals: first, to describe the theory behind each research demonstration project; and, second, to discuss the process of implementing the experimental intervention within the unique circumstances of each site. In considering whether to develop this compendium of intervention strategies, there was some concern over whether to describe the projects before we knew how successful they were. The consensus of the participating sites, however, was to present these descriptions for at least the following two reasons.

First, each proposed program was based on some prior experience and theoretical rationale. A description of this logic might be helpful to others considering program design and might offer new ideas to those with existing programs. In many cases, given the current state-of-the-art, these are our best guesses of what types of programming are likely to be successful.

Secondly, few journals publishing the results of experimental evalua-

[Haworth co-indexing entry note]: "Introduction." Conrad, Kendon J., Cheryl I. Hultman, and John S. Lyons. Co-published simultaneously in the *Alcoholism Treatment Quarterly* (The Haworth Press, Inc.) Vol. 10, No. 3/4, 1993, pp. 1-4; and: *Treatment of the Chemically Dependent Homeless: Theory and Implementation in Fourteen American Projects* (ed: Kendon J. Conrad, Cheryl I. Hultman, and John S. Lyons) The Haworth Press, Inc., 1993, pp. 1-4. Multiple copies of this article/chapter may be purchased from The Haworth Document Delivery Center [1-800-3-HAWORTH: 9:00 a.m. - 5:00 p.m. (EST)].

tions of demonstration projects have the space to allow for detailed discussion of program theory, design and implementation that has been afforded in the present volume. As these chapters show, a great deal was learned about implementing innovative programming for the homeless with substance abuse disorders. This volume documents these important efforts as well as the resulting, modified interventions. Future research evaluating the effectiveness of these projects can now refer to this document so that program planners and researchers are better informed about the complex nature of the various experimental interventions.

OVERVIEW

The first chapter is an overview of the NIAAA Cooperative Agreement by Huebner, Perl, Murray, Scott, and Tutunjian, all of whom are staff members of the NIAAA Homeless Demonstration and Evaluation Branch that directed this innovative collaborative approach to research and service provision. This chapter presents important background information and a description of the ground rules that form a foundation for understanding the subsequent chapters.

Each of these chapters, like the projects themselves, is unique. However, most of them are organized to cover a common set of themes that all of the projects share. Each chapter includes a discussion of the setting of the program including descriptions of the political, economic, and social context in each city. The specific target population is described including its special needs. In most of the chapters, the customary services are described and compared with the innovative treatments, and the objectives of the proposed innovations are linked with the needs of the target population and the presumed gaps in customary services. This forms the theoretical rationale for believing that the program will be more effective than previously existing services.

After presenting the theoretical model, each chapter discusses some of the major issues that arose during implementation. Many of the projects share common themes such as: overcoming barriers at local, state, and federal levels; overcoming denial and motivating clients to begin treatment; selecting the most effective treatment alternatives and matching clients to treatment; residential care; relapse prevention strategies; intensive case management; employment and benefits acquisition and maintenance; and housing acquisition and maintenance.

In many cases, the fact that a researcher was designated by NIAAA to serve as principal investigator was a new situation for the program staff–a situation requiring some adjustment. Therefore, several of the chapters offer useful case studies of how research and clinical coalitions can work together to resolve control issues; work through the differences in training, goals and vocabulary, and resolve problems that arise due to the unusual demands of experimental research. Other chapters discuss the problems involved in implementing complex, multifaceted programs in a variety of economic, organizational, and political settings.

Along with the similarities, there was also a good deal of variation in program focus and design across the fourteen sites. For example, about half of the sites had an integrated residential component whereas the others did not. Instead, some sites offered enhanced day treatment programs with no residential care or intensive case management which was shelter-based. Some of the demonstrations were designed primarily for homeless men; some included women only; others included women and children. The St. Louis project for women and children actually involved two separate programs which are given separate chapters in this volume. Some programs were specifically designed for persons with co-existing psychiatric disorders. Others, while not including this case-mix characteristic in their program design, did not exclude participants with mental illness from their study sample.

It is in observing both the similarities and the differences that the potential for learning, based on the collective experiences of the fourteen sites, is the greatest. The similarities reveal the core programmatic issues on which there seems to be a great deal of consensus across projects. The differences indicate that projects are varying their approaches according to their special populations, situations, and philosophies.

ORGANIZATION OF THE BOOK

The book is organized in a fairly loose but logical sequence that follows the stages of program development. Whereas most of the chapters cover the topics discussed earlier, each of them highlights one or two aspects of program development somewhat more than the others. Some focus more heavily on general *theoretical* issues (Tucson, Chicago), while others have rich descriptions of the local *political* and social milieus (New Orleans, Newark, New Haven). Others emphasize the service needs of *special populations* such as women with children (St. Louis) or the dually diagnosed (Washington, D.C.). One chapter describes *outreach* strategies in great depth (Seattle), whereas another highlights *relapse and retention* issues (Philadelphia). Several chapters present thorough discussions of their *residential care* programs (Albuquerque, Evanston/VA, Los Angeles), whereas another focuses on its intensive *case management* techniques

(Denver). The *transition to independence* from supported residential programs to independent housing is the last major stage of program development that is emphasized (Birmingham). The final chapter of the book is a synthesis of some of our observations regarding some of the important features of the chapters with concluding discussions of the possible implications for future policy, practice and research.

ACKNOWLEDGMENTS

The co-editors would like to acknowledge the assistance and cooperation received from several different sources. Thomas McGovern, the Editor of the *Alcoholism Treatment Quarterly* (ATQ) was very supportive and helpful throughout the project. The national evaluation staff from NIAAA provided helpful suggestions on the introduction and synthesis. We are grateful to Robert Huebner, Ph.D., Acting Chief of the Homeless Demonstration and Evaluation Branch of NIAAA and Jack Scott, Sc.D., Operations Research Analyst from NIAAA; Robert Orwin, Ph.D., Research Director of R.O.W. Sciences; David Cordray, Ph.D., Professor of Public Policy and Psychology, and Georgine Pion, Ph.D., Research Associate Professor, both from the Vanderbilt Institute for Public Policy Studies. Finally, the Department of Veterans Affair's Midwest Health Services Research and Development Field Program provided generous administrative support for the production of this volume.

OVERVIEW
OF NIAAA COOPERATIVE
AGREEMENT PROGRAM

The NIAAA Cooperative
Agreement Program for Homeless Persons
with Alcohol and Other Drug Problems:
An Overview

Robert B. Huebner, PhD
Harold I. Perl, PhD
Peggy M. Murray, MSW
Jack E. Scott, ScD
Beth Ann Tutunjian, MPH

Robert B. Huebner, Harold I. Perl, Peggy M. Murray, Jack E. Scott, and Beth Ann Tutunjian are on staff in the Homeless Demonstration and Evaluation Branch, Division of Clinical and Prevention Research, National Institute on Alcohol Abuse and Alcoholism, Room 13C-06, 5600 Fishers Lane, Rockville, MD 20857.

The authors would like to acknowledge the contribution of Robert G. Orwin, L. Joseph Sonnefeld, and Roberta Garrison of ROW Sciences, Inc. and David Cordray and Georgine Pion of Vanderbilt University.

[Haworth co-indexing entry note]: "The NIAAA Cooperative Agreement Program for Homeless Persons with Alcohol and Other Drug Problems: An Overview." Huebner, Robert B. et al. Co-published simultaneously in the *Alcoholism Treatment Quarterly* (The Haworth Press, Inc.) Vol. 10, No. 3/4, 1993, pp. 5-20; and *Treatment of the Chemically Dependent Homeless: Theory and Implementation in Fourteen American Projects* (ed: Kendon J. Conrad, Cheryl I. Hultman, and John S. Lyons) The Haworth Press, Inc., 1993, pp. 5-20. Multiple copies of this article/chapter may be purchased from The Haworth Document Delivery Center [1-800-3-HAWORTH: 9:00 a.m. - 5:00 p.m. (EST)].

SUMMARY. Alcohol and other drug abuse represent the most predominant public health problem facing the nation's growing homeless population. Few treatment services are available for homeless persons with alcohol or other drug abuse problems, and little is known about the effectiveness of these services. In 1990, the National Institute on Alcohol Abuse and Alcoholism (NIAAA) launched a three-year, fourteen-project research demonstration program to develop, implement, and evaluate the effectiveness of treatment interventions for this target population. This article describes the background, goals, and structure of the NIAAA Cooperative Agreement Program.[1]

INTRODUCTION

Over the last decade, it has become increasingly apparent to researchers and service providers alike that a significant segment of the nation's contemporary homeless population experiences severe and chronic problems with alcohol and other drugs. Although precise national estimates are unavailable, the prevalence of current alcohol abuse and dependence among the homeless population in the United States is approximately 45 percent and an additional 30 percent of the homeless population abuses other drugs (Lehman & Cordray, in press). Moreover, evidence suggests that the problems of alcohol and other drug abuse and homelessness cut across a wider range of sociodemographic groups than in the past. In the 1940s and 1950s, homeless persons with alcohol problems were primarily older, white males who lived in the nation's urban centers or "skid rows" (Garrett, 1989; Rossi, 1989). Recent epidemiologic surveys of homeless persons, however, have found alcohol and other drug abuse problems among women, minorities, young men, and increasing numbers of youth (Fisher, 1991; Robertson, Koegel & Ferguson, 1989). The National Academy of Sciences has concluded that alcohol and other drug abuse represents the most predominant public health problem for persons who are homeless (Institute of Medicine, 1988).

THE FEDERAL RESPONSE TO HOMELESSNESS

In the 1980s the plight of homeless people began to receive national attention. Early efforts by the U.S. Congress focused on emergency food and shelter administered through the Federal Emergency Management Agency (FEMA) and emergency shelter and transitional housing programs run by the Department of Housing and Urban Development (HUD). The first major omnibus legislative response to homelessness came in July

of 1987 with the passage of the Stewart B. McKinney Home
tance Act. An important feature of this legislation was that it w
the "emergency" response to create twenty new programs ad
by seven federal agencies.

Among these programs were longer-term housing initiatives developed
by HUD, such as the Section 8 Moderate Rehabilitation Program, as well
as housing programs that provided services for special needs populations,
including homeless people with serious mental illness or physical handi-
caps. Most importantly, the McKinney Act recognized that homeless individuals have needs that extend beyond housing. Funds were provided to
the Department of Education to develop education and literacy programs for
homeless adults and children. The Department of Labor was given authority
to develop and evaluate job training programs for homeless individuals.
Chronically mentally ill homeless veterans were targeted to receive services
through special Department of Veteran's Affairs programs. And finally, the
Department of Health and Human Services was given authority to administer five programs that focused on the primary health, mental health, and
alcohol and other drug treatment needs of homeless individuals and families. One element of the federal response, Section 613 of the McKinney Act,
authorized funds for the National Institute on Alcohol Abuse and Alcoholism (NIAAA) to support a demonstration program to develop, implement,
and evaluate innovative treatment interventions for homeless individuals
with alcohol and other drug abuse problems.

COMMUNITY DEMONSTRATION PROGRAM

In May 1988, NIAAA initiated the Community Demonstration Projects
for Alcohol and Other Drug Abuse Treatment of Homeless Individuals
(hereinafter referred to as the Community Demonstration program). This
program awarded a total of $9.2 million for two-year grants to nine com-
munity-based projects in eight cities: Anchorage, AK; Boston, MA; Los
Angeles, CA; Louisville, KY; Minneapolis, MN; New York, NY; Oakland,
CA; and two projects in Philadelphia, PA. Seven of the original nine
projects were awarded a total of $4.5 million for a third year which con-
cluded in September 1991.

The structure of this demonstration program was distinctive in two
important ways. First, NIAAA purposely did *not* prescribe a single, uniform treatment protocol to be implemented and evaluated. This decision
was based on the fact that little empirical knowledge existed regarding
what types of treatments were effective with homeless persons. Applicants
were free to choose the nature and scope of the intervention models to be

investigated, resulting in the eventual funding of a rich mix of treatment approaches rather than the demonstration of a single model in different settings.

A second distinctive feature of the Community Demonstration program was its emphasis on evaluation. The Request for Applications (RFA) required that each grantee (1) allocate at least 25 percent of the award for evaluation purposes; (2) conduct a process evaluation of the project; and (3) participate in a national evaluation of the full demonstration program. In addition, applicants were encouraged, though not required, to conduct evaluations of the impact of proposed interventions on individual clients. Seven of the nine projects attempted to assess the impact of program interventions using experimental or quasi-experimental designs. In addition to site-specific instruments of their own choosing, each used the *Addiction Severity Index* (ASI) (McLellan, Luborsky, Cacciola, McGahan, & O'Brien, 1988) to measure outcomes related to employment and support status, alcohol and other drug use, family/social relationships, medical and psychiatric conditions, and legal status. The ASI provided the national evaluators with standardized data with which to assess outcomes across sites.

The Community Demonstration Program broke new ground in a number of ways. The program was the first to support comprehensive interventions that were designed specifically to treat homeless people with alcohol and other drug problems. A variety of innovative approaches to serving the target population were developed, such as outreach to streets and homeless shelters, intensive case management, and educational and vocational training programs. A detailed description of these interventions can be found in a special issue of *Alcoholism Treatment Quarterly* (Argeriou & McCarty, 1990). Also, for the first time a significant attempt was made to support services while learning as much as possible about the nature and impact of those services. The direct funding of treatment programs *and* the requirements to devote a significant portion of those funds for evaluation reflects this dual purpose. Finally, this demonstration program developed a number of strategies to overcome the methodological challenges that emerged in developing a multi-site evaluation of this type (Huebner & Crosse, 1991).

Lessons Learned in the Community Demonstration Program

The Community Demonstration program yielded many valuable lessons in designing multi-site research demonstration projects. One critical lesson was the importance of allowing time for project start up–especially for service providers who are developing new interventions. Even those projects that were thoroughly planned and well conceptualized met with significant barriers to implementation. In fact, several projects, most notably those proposing residential components, took more than a full year to become operational. Another key lesson was the importance of requiring interventions to be of sufficient duration to allow for the collection of meaningful outcome data. Brief interventions (e.g., outreach) that involved only minimal contact with clients limited the amount of data that could be collected. It was found that these types of interventions needed to be linked with more extended interventions for purposes of evaluating program effects. A final lesson learned was that plans for tracking and follow up should be developed before the first client enters the program. These plans should also include gaining access to supplemental sources of data (e.g., administrative records), analytical plans for handling missing data when follow-up data are unavailable, and sensitivity analyses to determine the evaluation design's robustness to varying levels of client attrition.

COOPERATIVE AGREEMENT PROGRAM

In August 1990, NIAAA funded fourteen new projects in thirteen cities under the program of "Cooperative Agreements for Research Demonstration Projects on Alcohol and Other Drug Abuse Treatment for Homeless Persons" (hereinafter referred to as the Cooperative Agreement program). Figure 1 displays the location of these projects. The appropriation level for this three-year program was approximately $15.9 million in each of fiscal years 1990-1992. This program's mission was to support and to evaluate the effectiveness of interventions for homeless persons with alcohol and other drug problems. The primary goals of the program are to: (a) reduce the consumption of alcohol and other drugs; (b) increase levels of shelter and residential stability; and (c) enhance the participants' economic or employment status. The secondary goals of the program are to improve the participants' health and mental health status and to increase cooperation and linkages among community-based service agencies addressing the needs of homeless persons.

The Cooperative Agreement program has a number of unique features that were intended to sharpen how services were conceptualized and to increase the methodological rigor of the demonstration program at both the project and national level. One very significant feature was the choice of funding mechanism. NIAAA awarded cooperative agreements instead of grants because the former mechanism provided for the substantial involvement of NIAAA staff in the management and evaluation of the projects. Thus, the current program allowed individual applicants to develop their

Figure 1
Location of Project Sites in NIAAA Cooperative Agreement Program

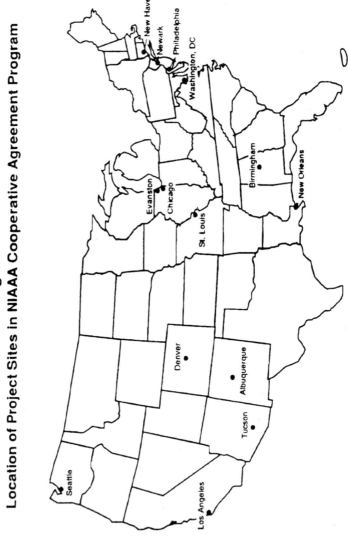

own interventions and research hypotheses, while providing NIAAA staff with the opportunity to obtain common data *across* sites for national-level and multi-site reports.

Developing Guidelines for Service Interventions

The guidelines for the development of service interventions were crafted to encourage creative combinations of treatment interventions. Two broad categories were established as parameters in constructing a program: *initial* interventions and *extended* interventions. Initial interventions were defined as activities aimed toward stabilizing clients and then linking them with treatment that was long-term in nature. Examples of such activities are outreach, detoxification and sobering services. Extended interventions normally occur post-stabilization and include such activities as case management, alcohol and drug treatment, self-help, housing, and vocational training services. Funding was available for the support of either one or more extended services *or* an initial intervention linked with an extended intervention. As discussed earlier, one key lesson from the Community Demonstration program was that initial interventions with no long-term contact severely constrained the amount and quality of data that could be obtained for the evaluation of programs.

Developing Guidelines for Site-Level Evaluations

A major consideration in planning the Cooperative Agreement program was to build in the capability to answer questions about program efficacy in the most scientifically rigorous manner possible. Similar to the Community Demonstration program, each grantee was required to devote at least 25 percent of grant funds to evaluation activities, conduct a process evaluation, and participate in the national, multi-site evaluation. A critical additional requirement was that each grantee was directed to conduct a client-level outcome evaluation of their intervention.

The essential components of the mandated process evaluation were that the evaluation data be quantitative, longitudinal, and collected on the individual level. At a minimum, these evaluation data were expected to answer questions about the characteristics of clients, the organization of the intervention, implementation history, and the treatment status of clients. Additional data on initial interventions could be collected and reported on an aggregate level. Applicants were encouraged to collect other types of process data on the operation of their program (e.g., costs of services).

Although the outcome evaluation was required, its parameters were broad: applicants were required to establish one or more comparison groups and administer a core set of instruments compiled by NIAAA (described below) at specified points in time (i.e., intake, discharge, and six months post-discharge). Applicants were also encouraged to develop other measures of program impact and use multiple methods where possible. These requirements ensured that each proposed intervention would have a fair and strong test of its effectiveness, yet gave applicants flexibility in the development of an evaluation design.

DESIGNING THE NATIONAL EVALUATION

The national, multi-site evaluation has three primary purposes: (1) to develop an in-depth profile of homeless persons with alcohol and other drug abuse problems; (2) to improve the knowledge base regarding the effectiveness of interventions for this target population; and (3) to compare outcomes, where possible, across different types of interventions and communities. Consequently, the national evaluation is designed to yield information and inferences that may be impossible to glean from an individual site-level assessment. It builds upon the site-level evaluations in such a way that it has the advantages of a depth of focus that can only come with intimate, site-level understanding of an intervention as well as a broadness of view that comes from a perspective of multiple interventions across multiple sites.

The national, multi-site evaluation is comprised of four key components: the logic models that describe the steps of the interventions and the theoretical rationale for their expected effectiveness; the core battery of standard instruments mandated by NIAAA; two measures of service provision that were developed by the national evaluation team[2] in collaboration with the Cooperative Agreement investigators; and the project-developed assessments of project implementation and linkages to local service systems.

Logic Models

Sets of logic models, literally graphic displays of each intervention's goals, specific activities, anticipated outcomes, and theoretical rationales for change, have been developed for each project site. They identify the key components of the intervention, their implementation and operation, and their inevitable evolution over time. A phase-based series of logic models is under development: an initial model based on the intervention as it was originally proposed, one or more intermediate models based on the actual implementation of the various intervention components at successive points in time, and, eventually, one model which will represent the most comprehensively operational version of the intervention.

Core Battery of Instruments

Each Cooperative Agreement project was required to administer a core battery of standard assessment instruments specified by NIAAA to collect individual-level outcome evaluation data on all study participants in the intervention and control conditions. This battery consists of three instruments: the Addiction Severity Index (McLellan et al., 1988), the Alcohol Dependence Scale (Horn, Skinner, Wanberg & Foster, 1984), and the housing section of the Personal History Form (Barrow, Hellman, Lovell, Plapinger, Robinson & Struening, 1985). These are described below.

Addiction Severity Index (ASI): The ASI is a structured, 45-minute clinical research instrument designed to assess problem severity in seven domains that are often critical for persons with alcohol and other drug problems: alcohol use, drug use, employment, family relations, illegal activities, medical condition, and psychiatric condition. For each of the domains, objective questions are asked that measure the number, extent and duration of problem symptoms in the patient's lifetime or over the past 30 days.

Alcohol Dependence Scale (ADS): The ADS is a 25-item, forced-choice instrument which is administered in an interview format at baseline only for this program, taking approximately five minutes to complete. It was developed to provide a brief measure of alcohol dependence syndrome. A cardinal element of this syndrome is the extent to which a person manifests impaired control over alcohol intake. Other aspects include severe alcohol withdrawal symptoms, awareness of a compulsion to drink excessively, increased tolerance to alcohol, and salience of drink-seeking behavior.

Personal History Form (PHF): The PHF is a survey form that was developed specifically for recording information about homeless persons. The Cooperative Agreement Program utilizes only the residential history section of the PHF, which contains 34 items that document the respondent's lifetime residence history including episodes of homelessness.

Each of the three instruments was originally designed for use with a population other than that of homeless persons with alcohol and drug problems. Consequently, the national evaluation team sought to improve the quality of data that would flow from these instruments by revising their content and structure so that they would be more appropriate to the program's participants. These revisions were made in close consultation and collaboration with the principal investigators in the Cooperative Agreement projects, the investigators who used similar instruments in the earlier Community Demonstration program, and the authors of the instruments themselves. At the present time, the national evaluation team and investigators from the individual sites are conducting studies to determine the reliability and validity characteristics of the revised instrument protocols.

Measuring Services

The Cooperative Agreement program utilizes two major data sources for information regarding the level and intensity of services that the program participants receive: the Quarterly Report Form (QRF) and the Treatment Services Interview (TSI). The QRF was designed and developed by the national evaluation team, in collaboration with the Cooperative Agreement principal investigators and in consultation with an expert panel. The foundation of the QRF is the *Glossary of Service Activities for Alcohol and Other Drug Abuse Treatment of Homeless Persons* (NIAAA, 1991) which defines 39 specific services that can be provided in various community and institutional settings. The QRF combines these service types and settings to form a matrix which can describe whether a particular client receives a particular service in a particular setting. The matrix also designates the provider of the service (e.g., case manager, addictions counselor). Finally, the QRF collects data on program implementation, funding source, client flow, and system linkage with other service providers. For the purposes of this program, the QRF collects data only on the use of services provided by agencies directly affiliated with a Cooperative Agreement project. The Treatment Services Interview (TSI) was developed by the national evaluation team and the Cooperative Agreement principal investigators to serve as an adjunct to the QRF. The TSI is a brief client self-report interview form that is designed to assess the client's use of treatment services from all sources during the preceding 60 days.

Program Implementation and Systems Level Activities

The documentation of program implementation history and activities at the systems level is another key component of the national, multi-site evaluation. In fact, one of the research objectives of the Cooperative Agreement program is to increase levels of cooperation and linkage among service agencies that address the needs of homeless persons with alcohol and other drug problems. NIAAA has developed several methods to obtain useful data regarding program implementation and systems level activities.

Information regarding program implementation, including both the barriers to success and the steps taken to counteract them, is obtained from several sources. Among these are the logic models described above, data from the QRF, bimonthly telephone consultations held by national evaluation staff with project-level staff at every site, and annual site visits to each project. The logic models provide a graphic display of the various components of the intervention as they are actually configured at any particular time. The QRF provides narrative data on the status of program implementation and systems linkage activities. Similar information regarding systems level activities by the project are obtained from the bimonthly phone calls, the on-site visits, and the QRF.

SYNTHESIS OF THE COOPERATIVE AGREEMENT PROJECTS

As can be seen in Table 1, the projects in the Cooperative Agreement program reflect a great deal of diversity in terms of target populations, types of interventions, and evaluation designs. Over 6,000 homeless persons, predominantly minority men, are anticipated to be served in this research demonstration program. Nine of the original fourteen projects serve both men and women, one project offers services for women with children, two projects focus on homeless persons with a chronic mental illness concomitant with a substance abuse problem, and one project serves veterans exclusively.

Specific service components demonstrated in this program include outreach, detoxification, psychotherapy, self-help groups, vocational training, and family counseling. Three broad categories of services have emerged: case management, recovery and treatment programs, and housing services. Thirteen of the projects provide some form of case management, ten provide recovery and treatment services, and ten provide housing services. Those projects that do not provide treatment or housing services themselves utilize existing community resources. (A more complete synthesis of the fourteen projects can be found in the plan for the national, multi-site evaluation [R.O.W. Sciences, Inc. & Vanderbilt Institute for Public Policy Studies, 1990], while detailed descriptions of the projects themselves appear in other chapters of this volume.)

Although case management is clearly the most common service type provided across the projects, a variety of different case management models are being implemented. For example, Denver, Philadelphia, and Seattle provide direct case management and link clients to *existing* community-

Table 1. Descriptions of Projects in NIAAA Cooperative Agreement Program

Project Name	Treatment Setting	Service Interventions and Evaluation Designs
Albuquerque, NM	Community-based detoxification center, transitional alcohol- and drug-free housing	Residential detoxification, then random assignment to one of three groups: (1) high-intensity services group receiving supervised transitional housing, case management, and case manager-facilitated alcohol and other drug treatment; (2) medium-intensity group receiving supervised transitional housing but only self-initiated treatment; (3) low-intensity group receiving self-initiated treatment (some clients in this group received individual housing).
Birmingham, AL	Outpatient clinic, community center	Random assignment to one of two groups: (1) intensive outpatient intervention that includes daily alcohol and other drug treatment sessions and aftercare program; (2) usual care.
Chicago, IL	Community service agency, supportive housing	Random assignment to one of three groups: (1) intensive case management plus supportive housing; (2) intensive case management only; (3) control.
Denver, CO	Alcohol and other drug treatment agency, transitional housing	Intensive community outreach program, then random assignment to one of two groups: (1) usual treatment plus intensive case management; (2) usual treatment only.
Evanston, IL	VA hospital	Random assignment to one of two groups: (1) case-managed residential care; (2) usual treatment in current VA alcohol and other drug treatment unit.
Los Angeles, CA	Community-based socialization center, residential treatment facility	Random assignment to one of three groups: (1) treatment in a non-residential program; (2) treatment through a new service linkage with an existing residential treatment program; (3) existing day socialization program.
New Haven, CT	Monitored shelter, community agencies	Random assignment to one of two groups: (1) alcohol and other drug treatment and intensive case management in a closely monitored drug-free shelter; (2) limited case management in drug-free but unmonitored shelters.

New Orleans, LA	Social detoxification facility, monitored housing units	Social detoxification then random assignment to one of two groups: (1) usual care; (2) transitional housing with possible continuation at extended residential alcohol and other drug treatment facility with intensive case management.
Newark, NJ	Hospital outpatient clinic, alcohol- and drug-free transitional housing, vocational training center	Random assignment to one of two groups: (1) on-site case management plus vocational training; (2) standard public welfare case management.
Philadelphia, PA	Shelter, alcohol and other drug treatment facility, transitional housing facility	Random assignment to one of three groups: (1) supervised housing and case management integrated with alcohol and other drug treatment and vocational/educational services; (2) monitored shelter and intensive case management with a community-based network of services; (3) typical shelter services with usual casework.
Seattle, WA	County-operated detoxification facility	Random assignment to one of two groups: (1) long-term intensive case management; (2) treatment as usual.
St. Louis, MO	Family shelters, supervised transitional housing facility	Random assignment to one of six groups. Four groups are housed at two Salvation Army shelters and also receive one of the following: (1) usual care; (2) extended case management; (3) family services intervention; (4) both extended case management and family services intervention. Remaining two groups receive intensive outpatient treatment and multiple support services while residing either in: (1) supervised alcohol- and drug-free residential facility; (2) existing shelters.
Tucson, AZ	Non-residential center, residential therapeutic community	Random assignment to one of two groups: (1) non-residential counseling, educational, and socialization center; (2) modified residential therapeutic community linked with community-based network of services.
Washington, DC	Private mental health agency, transitional housing	Random assignment to one of two models of intensive case management: (1) case managers provide treatment for both mental health and alcohol and other drug issues along with long term transitional housing; (2) case managers provide mental health services only, link clients to other alcohol and drug services, and work to restructure clients' social support networks.

based housing and recovery services. The remaining projects provide case management as an adjunct to outpatient or residential alcohol and drug treatment or with alcohol or drug free housing. In these instances, the case manager has the combined responsibility of providing case management services as well as alcohol and drug treatment. The caseloads of case managers across the projects range from 2 to 38, with a mode of 15.

Alcohol and other drug treatment and recovery services are provided by ten of the fourteen projects. These include individual and group counseling, educational programs on alcohol and other drugs, and participation in self-help groups such as Alcoholics Anonymous. These treatment and recovery services also vary in terms of their frequency, duration and counselor/client ratio. For example, treatment duration ranges from three to eighteen months while the modal value for counselor/client ratio was 1:15.

Housing services are also a key element across the demonstration projects. Ten projects provide either transitional or permanent housing services. About half of these are shelter-type settings and nine projects provide housing that is alcohol- and drug-free. Many projects offer supportive services as part of their housing component including alcohol and drug abuse recovery services and self-help groups. Finally, seven projects also offer permanent housing assistance which may include expert staff assistance, financial aid, the direct provision of permanent housing or linkage with community resources to develop additional housing options.

THE NIAAA DISSEMINATION STRATEGY

The final aspect of the NIAAA Cooperative Agreement and Community Demonstration programs is the development of a broad knowledge base regarding alcohol and drug abuse services for homeless people. A substantial amount of information will be generated regarding the challenges and accomplishments in the implementation of these innovative programs, the factors associated with clients' completion or non-completion of the treatment, and the effectiveness of these interventions on homeless persons' alcohol and other drug use, employment patterns, residential stability, and health and mental health status. Moreover, much will be learned about the limitations and lessons of conducting multi-site research demonstrations in general, as well as those regarding this vulnerable segment of the homeless population, in particular.

Dissemination of this knowledge is a priority for NIAAA. Findings from the Cooperative Agreement program will be disseminated through a range of formats and methods which target a wide audience that includes policy makers, service providers, and researchers. The NIAAA Homeless

Demonstration and Evaluation Branch has been active in providing information to the service and research communities since 1988. The Branch publishes technical assistance papers, process and outcome evaluation reports, and periodic program communiques. Branch staff members make frequent presentations at conferences and professional meetings. The Branch also maintains a dedicated mailing list that includes over 1,500 individuals in the fields of homelessness, alcohol and other drug treatment to disseminate information through the National Clearinghouse on Alcohol and Drug Information (NCADI). These dissemination activities are a critical component to NIAAA's research demonstration for homeless persons and will continue to provide state-of-the-art information to a wide audience on alcohol and other drug treatment for homeless persons.

AUTHOR NOTES

1. The formal title of this research demonstration program is "Cooperative Agreements for Research Demonstration Projects on Alcohol and Other Drug Abuse Treatment for Homeless Persons." The demonstration program was conducted in consultation with the National Institute on Drug Abuse (NIDA).

2. The national evaluation team for the Cooperative Agreement Program consisted of the following individuals: David S. Cordray, Georgine Pion (Vanderbilt University); Robert G. Orwin, L. Joseph Sonnefeld, Roberta Garrison, Jo-Ann Lucchese, Margaret Blasinsky, Mary Lou Jacobs, Stephanie Chesnutt, and Anne Sherman (ROW Sciences); Howard Goldman (University of Maryland); Robert B. Huebner, Harold I. Perl, and Jack E. Scott (NIAAA).

REFERENCES

Argeriou, M. & McCarty, D. (Eds.). (1990). Treating alcoholism and drug abuse among homeless men and women: nine community demonstration grants [Special Issue]. *Alcoholism Treatment Quarterly, 7*(1).

Barrow, S.M., Hellman, F., Lovell, A.M., Plapinger, J.D., Robinson, C.R., & Struening, E.L. (1985). *Personal History Form.* New York: New York State Psychiatric Institute.

Fischer, P. (1991). *Alcohol, Drug Abuse and Mental Health Problems Among Homeless Persons: A Review of the Literature 1980-1990.* Rockville, MD: U.S. Department of Health and Human Services.

Garrett, G.R. (1989). Alcohol problems and homelessness: history and research. *Contemporary Drug Problems, 1989, 16*(3), 301-332.

Horn, J.L., Skinner, H.A., Wanberg, K., & Foster, F.M. (1984). *Alcohol Dependence Scale (ADS).* Toronto: Addiction Research Foundation of Ontario.

Huebner, R.B., & Crosse, S.B. (1991). Challenges in evaluating a national demonstration program for homeless persons with alcohol and other drug problems. *New Directions for Program Evaluation, 52*(4), 33-46.

Institute of Medicine. (1988). *Homelessness, Health, and Human Needs.* Washington, DC: National Academy Press.

Lehman, A.F. & Cordray, D.S. (in press). Prevalence of alcohol, drug, and mental disorders among the homeless: One more time. *Contemporary Drug Problems.*

McLellan, A.T., Luborsky, L., Cacciola, J., McGahan, P., & O'Brien, C.P. (1988). *Guide to the Addiction Severity Index: Background, Administration, and Field Testing Results.* Washington, D.C.: National Institute on Drug Abuse.

Robertson, M.J., Koegel, P., & Ferguson, L. (1989). Alcohol use and abuse among homeless adolescents in Hollywood. *Contemporary Drug Problems, 16*(3), 415-452.

Rossi, P.H. (1990). The old homeless and the new homeless in historical perspective. *American Psychologist, 45,* 954-959.

R.O.W. Sciences, Inc. & Vanderbilt Institute for Public Policy Studies (1990). *Final National Evaluation Plan* (Contract No. ADM 281-90-0003). Rockville, MD: National Institute on Alcohol Abuse and Alcoholism.

THEORETICAL ISSUES: TUCSON, CHICAGO

A Therapeutic Community Model for Treatment of Homeless Alcohol and Drug Users in Tucson, Arizona

Sally J. Stevens, PhD
Julie Reed Erickson, PhD
Jarrie Carnell Tent
Jenny Chong, PhD
Philip Gianas

SUMMARY. The Amity Settlement Services for Education and Transition (ASSET) project was implemented in response to the

Sally J. Stevens, Jarrie Carnell Tent, and Philip Gianas are affiliated with Amity, Inc. Julie Reed Erickson and Jenny Chong are affiliated with the University of Arizona, College of Medicine.

Address correspondence to: Dr. Sally J. Stevens, Director of Research, Amity, Inc., 47 E. Pennington, Tucson, AZ 85701.

This project is funded by the National Institute of Alcohol Abuse and Alcoholism, 1 U01 AA08788.

[Haworth co-indexing entry note]: "A Therapeutic Community Model for Treatment of Homeless Alcohol and Drug Users in Tucson, Arizona." Stevens, Sally J. et al. Co-published simultaneously in the *Alcoholism Treatment Quarterly* (The Haworth Press, Inc.) Vol. 10, No. 3/4, 1993, pp. 21-33; and: *Treatment of the Chemically Dependent Homeless: Theory and Implementation in Fourteen American Projects* (ed: Kendon J. Conrad, Cheryl I. Hultman, and John S. Lyons) The Haworth Press, Inc., 1993, pp. 21-33. Multiple copies of this article/chapter may be purchased from The Haworth Document Delivery Center [1-800-3-HAWORTH: 9:00 a.m. - 5:00 p.m. (EST)].

21

needs of homeless substance abusing adults in Tucson, Arizona. The ASSET project used a modified therapeutic community model to address issues of (1) substance abuse, (2) homelessness, (3) employment and (4) health. This paper describes the target population, the objectives of the project, and the theoretical foundations of the treatment. Practical issues, problems in implementation and implications for future research demonstration projects are discussed.

AMITY SETTLEMENT SERVICES FOR EDUCATION AND TRANSITION

The Amity Settlement Services for Education and Transition (ASSET) project is a joint project of Amity, Incorporated and the University of Arizona, College of Medicine. The intervention component of the ASSET project is coordinated by Amity. Amity is a therapeutic community which provides substance abuse treatment for many different populations including juveniles and adults, adults on probation, incarcerated juveniles and adults, mothers and children and homeless. The research component of the ASSET project is coordinated by the University of Arizona, College of Medicine. The collaboration between Amity and the College of Medicine on research issues such as alcohol and drug treatment and AIDS prevention has been ongoing since 1987.

Background and Significance

The homeless population in Tucson, Arizona is reflective of the findings from studies conducted in other cities in the United States in terms of the multiple interrelated needs of the homeless population. These needs, however, are complicated by the fact that a great proportion of the homeless adults in Tucson have (1) come from different areas of the United States, and (2) exhibit extensive alcohol and/or drug problems. Erickson, Estrada and Stevens (1992) report a highly mobile drug abusing population in Tucson. Many of the transient adults have originally moved from the east coast or southern United States to Tucson. Without extended family support, these adults are left on their own to resettle. There is no family to accommodate them with bathing facilities, change of clothes, telephone or a mailing address. Without these accommodations, obtaining employment becomes difficult. Employment opportunities are further hindered by the fact that Tucson exhibits a high unemployment rate. Eventually, many of these adults end up in one of the Tucson shelters for the homeless (Bissell, 1992). Public services such as vocational training, housing and health care can be difficult to access. Without guidance from family members or friends who know the "system," a homeless adult may never problem solve the route to obtaining and utilizing these public services.

Estimates of homeless adults in Tucson who evidence alcohol and drug problems range from 40 to 60%. One reason for this high estimate is the ease with which drugs and alcohol can be obtained. The Arizona/Mexico border provides a corridor for large amounts of high quality, inexpensive drugs. Many of these drugs are highly addictive (e.g., heroin, cocaine). As Tucson, Arizona is the first major metropolitan area north of the border, many of the drugs are brought to Tucson. Due to the easy accessibility of drugs and alcohol, homeless people are frequently exposed to open drug and alcohol use in parks, public areas, shelters, etc. Gateway Larc, a detoxification center in Tucson, reports that approximately 90% of their clients are homeless and over 90% are being detoxed for a combination of alcohol and cocaine (McNamara, 1992).

Along with alcohol and drug abuse, lack of adequate housing and lack of employment, the homeless adults in Tucson, Arizona experience numerous health problems. El Rio Health Clinic, which is only one of the clinics that serves the homeless, reports that over 5,000 health/medical issues are documented for homeless adults each year for the Tucson metropolitan area alone (Black, 1992). While many of these cases are one time admissions, the majority represent homeless adults with multiple health problems.

Objectives of Treatment

The ASSET project is funded by the National Institute of Alcohol Abuse and Alcoholism (NIAAA) and is one of several research demonstration grants nationwide. Objectives of the ASSET project are similar to those of some of the other collaborating projects. Given the number of homeless, unemployed adults in Tucson who exhibit alcohol, drug, and other health problems, the ASSET project attempts to address four treatment objectives. These objectives include:

1. To reduce alcohol/drug use
2. To increase residential stability
3. To improve personal health
4. To improve employment capabilities/employment status

Theory of Treatment

One model for treatment which appears promising is that of the therapeutic community (TC). The TC prototype is ancient, existing in all forms of communal healing and support. The TC for substance abuse emerged in the 1960s as a self-help alternative to existing conventional treatments and was first applied to the treatment of male heroin addicts (Rom-Rymer, 1981). The foundations or roots of the TC are not from a medical model approach, but rather are based in the tradition of the Alcoholics Anonymous Twelve Step Self-Help Model. *TC's provide a microcosm of society in which people who have problems with alcohol, drugs and other alienating behaviors can learn to deal with the many facets which have driven their behavior.* In examining the effectiveness of the TC, Condelli and Danteman (in press) demonstrate that therapeutic communities are powerful interventions that even overshadow client variables when predicting retention and success. As the TC movement grew, the methodologies used and services provided were expanded and adapted to meet the special needs of a number of typically underserved populations. Besides adult substance abusers, groups receiving treatment in the TC model since the 1960s most often include (1) those with criminal justice involvement, and (2) those with co-morbidity issues (DeLeon, 1988). Other populations that have received less attention include adolescents, ethnic minorities, women and children and the homeless (Stevens & Glider, in press).

Most TC's, no matter what sub-population of addicted people they serve, accept that the principal aim of the TC is a global change in lifestyle including abstinence from illicit substances, elimination of antisocial behavior, and evidence of employability, prosocial attitudes and values (DeLeon, 1986). To achieve this aim, it has been thought that long term 15-24 months of treatment is necessary. Research efforts that examine length of stay or retention rates demonstrate a positive correlation between length of stay and success. In spite of this evidence, several investigators have demonstrated client success with shorter treatment durations. Glider et al. (in press) report success on a number of variables, i.e., a reduction in alcohol and drug use, criminal behavior and depression for inmates who participated in a TC jail program in which the average length of stay was approximately 4 months. Wexler, Falkin and Lipton (1990) report successful outcome data for a 6 month prison TC which served adult males with substance abuse problems. In examining data from the Drug Abuse Reporting Program (DARP) Simpson and Sells (1982) state that the minimum length of time in treatment to show positive treatment effect for a TC modality is about 3 months.

Whether the duration of the TC is four months or 24 months, the TC offers a systematic approach to achieving its principal aim. For the long-term TC, the treatment process can be outlined into phases. Mullen (1992) has outlined four phases for the long term residential TC at Amity, Inc. in

Tucson, Arizona. When participants first enter the TC, they participate in the *Basic Interface* curriculum for approximately 100 days. This first period is a time in which the individual can be assimilated into the community. The participant is assigned to a specific counselor who develops monthly treatment objectives and oversees the participant's progress. The participant is also assigned a senior resident to act as a "big brother." This "big brother" shares important information about day to day living and expectations in the TC and provides for an appropriate role model for the newcomer. The curriculum places a great deal of emphasis on changing one's life, being honest, making amends and taking responsibility. Constant and persistent participation is demanded.

When participants feel they are ready to move on, approval from both staff and other participants must be given. If approved, participants then join the *Community Class*. Curriculum during this second phase of the TC delves deeper into psychological and sociological issues. The curriculum is focused on moral development, personal discovery and family dynamics. Specific seminars are presented by staff and senior residents at least four times per week. Groups that address issues presented in the seminars as well as day to day living issues are held daily. At the Amity long-term residential TC, this phase is the longest; approximately 6 months. When a person feels ready to move on to the *Senior Class*, he/she makes a formal request and is given "Senior Questions" to address in writing. The written response is reviewed by both staff and peers and a community decision regarding the person's advancement is made.

The *Senior Class* is a time for the person to take on responsibility for the community. This is done by acting as a role model for newer members of the community and by assisting in the day to day operations of the facility. Additionally, it is a time for the individual to develop decision-making skills and plan for re-entry into the wider community.

Once the person moves out of the TC, it is expected that he/she maintain some ties to the TC by participating in *Continuance* or what has been traditionally known as "aftercare." This phase is not mandated but rather highly encouraged. Participants in *Continuance* offer support for one another while continuing with their own personal development.

Within each of the above outlined phases, there exist four concepts which must be provided for the participating adult to successfully and radically change his/her life (Mullen, 1992). These concepts include; (1) conflict, (2) sustained responsibility, (3) various roles, and (4) credible role models. TC's should challenge the participant's values and beliefs which have guided his/her past behavior. This challenge often creates a sense of conflict for the person. When a person comes into conflict with their originally held values and beliefs an opening for change occurs. This process can feel uncomfortable as it challenges the very essence of one's way of being. Oftentimes participants verbalize dislike for the program when this conflict is felt, yet as conflict is resolved a new perspective is evidenced.

Each day in the TC the participant must experience sustained responsibility. The participant must be held accountable for every behavior that he/she displays. Nothing must go unnoticed. All too often the addicted person has been able to walk away from responsibility, deny responsibility, numb responsibility with drugs, or rationalize why his/her behavior was the fault of someone else. Groups are held daily in which each person in the community can question another's behavior. As participants develop emotionally, intellectually, spiritually and physically, additional responsibilities, i.e., taking care of the facility and taking care of newcomers are added, thereby encouraging continual growth.

The TC model includes regular rituals such as daily morning and evening meetings, seminars, encounter groups, open houses, etc., in which everyone participates. These rituals are a way of manifesting shared values among participants and staff. Along with these rituals, it is important that people experience different "roles." At some point, a person may be asked to care for the newest members of the TC, host a meeting or seminar, work with the animals, or learn a completely new trade. Men are asked to take on roles often assumed by women and vice versa. At times the person is the student; at times the teacher. Taking on various roles provides for a sense of awareness of how others who are in those roles feel as well as a way to increase self awareness.

The TC provides credible role models who demonstrate the possibility of positive change in human life. The "newcomer" in the TC may not relate to the social worker or even a person who has been substance free for four or five years. Often one will hear the newcomer say "she is different from me" or "but he's been clean for five years." It is important that people involved in the recovery process have role models that make it a reality that dramatic positive change is possible. The TC environment provides for this role modeling, as some have been substance free for only a couple days while others have been drug free for years and have made tremendous positive changes in many areas of their lives. In a short period of time, the "newcomers" become a role model to others, pushing them to learn to hold themselves, as well as others, accountable. Self help, honesty and being one's brother or sister's keeper becomes the norm.

In the Tucson ASSET project these TC concepts are embraced. As a research demonstration project, the ASSET project utilizes the TC approach with a homeless substance abusing adult population. Since the TC model has proven effective for various populations of substance abusers, demonstration of success with the homeless would prove enlightening for both TC research and homeless research efforts. As outcome data from other TC programs that have used a three to six month length of stay have shown positive treatment effects, the Tucson ASSET project chose a 4-month program. Homeless adults were recruited to participate in the project. Those who agreed to participate were randomly assigned to either a residential or non-residential component. The four months of required involvement included a condensed version of phases 1, 2, and 3. Following the initial four month period, phase 4 was to be facilitated in a continuance setting. Recruited adults who did not wish to participate in the treatment portion of the project were asked to participate in a non-equivalent comparison group. Thus, this group provided a comparison between those who did not receive any treatment and the two treatment groups. Questions that the project staff were interested in answering in relationship to the treatment objectives included:

1. Does a modified TC approach work with homeless substance abusing adults?
2. If the approach does prove successful, what are the characteristics of the participants that it was successful for?
3. What aspects of the treatment process were particularly influential for that success to occur?
4. Can a TC approach be modified to a non-residential setting?
5. Can a shorter duration time (four months of formal enrolled treatment) prove effective?

HISTORY OF IMPLEMENTATION OF THE ASSET PROJECT

The history of the ASSET project began with an expressed need for such a program from a number of professionals directing or working with homeless substance abusing adults. An AIDS outreach and research project, COPASA, noted that approximately 20% of the injection drug users and their sexual partners that enrolled in the AIDS project were homeless. When facilitating referrals to treatment, COPASA staff found that services for the adult homeless substance abusing population were few and those that did offer treatment services often had lengthy waiting lists. Several meetings were then held with providers to assess accurately both services and gaps in services for this population. The end result of these meetings was a proposal to the National Institute of Alcohol Abuse and Alcoholism (NIAAA) for this research project. It was felt that a "research demonstration" proposal would be best in that many of the concepts to be tested were new. A strong research component would allow the project staff to fully evaluate the outcomes of the study.

The ASSET project began accepting participants into the project seven months after funding was awarded. Like most large new projects, barriers to implementation were experienced. The first major barrier in the implementation of the ASSET project was locating and securing a residential facility. Several houses large enough to accommodate 16-20 residents were located in two neighborhoods in Tucson. Being familiar with the "Not In My Backyard" (NIMBY) syndrome, project staff worked diligently to convince the neighbors that this project would not cause problems, but rather, may enhance the neighborhood. Door-to-door presentations were made, as well as formal presentations, at the neighborhood association meetings. This approach had some positive impact, as many neighbors agreed to accept the project. Yet the final vote was negative with one of the neighborhood associations reporting a 17 to 16 vote *not* in favor of ASSET.

Fortunately, project staff had initiated several attempts to locate housing simultaneously. Besides working with neighborhood associations, staff looked for residential sites not within zoning requirements. Another appropriate housing site in a third area of Tucson was located but it was not zoned for the purpose of the project. Therefore, a zoning variance for occupancy was filed with the Tucson Board of Adjustment.

Yet another route to housing acquisition involved negotiations with an already licensed house occupied by another project. After five and a half months into the first year, the latter two methods proved successful. As renovation and alterations were much less, occupancy could occur sooner in the housing facility negotiated from the other treatment project. Thus ASSET staff chose to secure that facility.

Projects planning to secure residential housing should work on several routes to acquisition of a facility at the same time. First, staff must understand zoning codes, revised statutes, fair housing laws and local ordinances. Secondly, staff should prepare their Board of Directors for a barrage of phone calls from concerned neighbors. Additionally, it is important to understand the specific powers of neighborhood associations. Oftentimes these associations wield strong political influence. Finally, be prepared to work within local government guidelines and anticipate at least six months of negotiations.

A second major barrier to implementation of the ASSET project was that the number of expected referrals from other treatment agencies, homeless shelters, the detoxification center and the county jail were less than expected. Several meetings occurred in advance with these agencies and preliminary assessments indicated that the number of referrals would be more than adequate for the project. Because this communication occurred in advance, little time was spent on participant recruitment from these agencies the first six months that the project was open. Realizing that recruitment of participants was a problem, ASSET staff again met with agency directors and then met directly with staff responsible for that agency's case management and referrals. Agency referrals to ASSET increased once the "on line" staff were educated about the ASSET project and knew the ASSET project staff personally. A second step to increase enrollment included the hiring of two outreach workers whose specific job assignment was that of recruitment. Besides working with referral agencies, the outreach workers conducted street outreach to parks, soup kitchens, and other areas where they could locate homeless adult men and women. Within two months of hiring the outreach workers, enrollment for the project increased dramatically.

It seems important to acknowledge that even in cities where homeless adults are numerous, one must not assume that enrollment will occur. Instead, a specific plan prior to the opening of the project should be developed and specific staff should be hired to be responsible for recruitment and enrollment activities. Furthermore, for recruitment to be successful one must involve staff from the referring agencies who work directly with the clients.

A third major barrier to implementation of the project was the tension that occurred between the research and intervention staff. Research demonstration projects add new dynamics that most service-only programs do not have. As approximately one quarter of the project staff are researchers, it is important that a positive working relationship develop between clinical staff and research staff. Goals of each team differ; the clinical team is more focused on development of the model and providing for the best possible service delivery. Often-times this requires flexibility in admission criteria, curriculum, program activities, and program design. The research team goals are to develop and *test* a model. This goal does not lend itself to flexibility. Because of the practical differences between approaches it is important that the teams understand the other's perspective. During the start-up period of the ASSET project the clinical and research teams met once per week for planning, cross training, and feedback. Because of direct talk, priorities were easier to set. In summary this time proved to be essential for the successful working relationship of the teams involved in the ASSET project.

A fourth issue which hindered project implementation was that of random assignment. Random assignment was a difficult concept for most of the clinical staff to accept. Often-times the particular life situation of a potential participant made him/her appear more appropriate for one component, thus making it difficult for the staff to accept that the assignment must be random. As the project moved forward, clinical staff became more comfortable with the random assignment and they learned how to verbally present both components to the potential participants as positive avenues for creating personal change. Emphasis was always placed on the ASSET project being a therapeutic and teaching community and not strictly a research project.

Descriptive Data

One hundred and sixty-five homeless adult men and women were enrolled in the Tucson ASSET project from April, 1991 through May, 1992. Demographic characteristics of the sample have been analyzed. Ninety percent of those who have enrolled in ASSET have been men while 10% have been women. The mean age for the ASSET participants is 34.7 years with 49% between the ages of 31 and 40 years of age. In terms of ethnicity, the general Tucson, Arizona population includes 69% White, 21% Hispanic, 4% Native American, 3% Black, and 3% other. During the first year of the ASSET project 63% of those enrolled were White, 9.7% Hispanic, 5.5% American Indian, 18.2% Black and 3.6% Asian/Pacific Islander or Other. When looking at veteran status for males only, 69% of the ASSET participants reported being a veteran.

Reasons for homelessness for the ASSET participants was assessed for both the first time that the person was homeless and the most recent time the person was homeless. Interestingly, for questions on "first time homeless" and "most recent homeless," most ASSET participants reported "alcohol/drug problems" as the reason (71% and 72% respectively). Other reasons most commonly mentioned were interpersonal conflict (39%; 27%), loss of job (37%; 31%), increased living expenses (26%; 18%), and benefactor unwilling to support (26%; 20%).

In examining drug use characteristics of homeless adults in the ASSET project, alcohol seems to be the most problematic with 63% of the enrollees reporting alcohol to be their most problematic drug. Cocaine/crack was second with 25% of the population reporting that this was their most programmatic drug. In terms of the drugs used within the last 30 days the most common drugs reported by ASSET participants at intake included alcohol, 89%; marijuana, 51%; and cocaine/crack, 40%.

As employment/employability was one of the four major treatment objectives of the project, employment status and patterns among ASSET participants were examined. Eighty-four percent of the ASSET participants reported having a profession, trade or skill. Most commonly reported types of professions included skilled manual labor (40%) and semi-skilled workers (16%). Interestingly, when length of longest full-time job was analyzed, 56% of the ASSET participants reported that their length of longest full-time job was between 1 and 5 years. Twenty-one percent reported less than one year while 15% reported 5 to 10 years. Seven percent reported that the length of longest full-time job was 11 to 20 years, while only 1% had never worked.

When looking at employment patterns in the past year, 33% of ASSET participants reported having full-time work, while 30% were unemployed. Regular and irregular part-time work was reported by 34% of the participants, while 3% were either a student, homemaker or were in a controlled environment. When questioned as to how many days they were paid for work in the last 30 days, 58% reported none, 32% reported 1-10, 8% reported 11-20, and 2% reported 21-30 days.

The health status of homeless adults is also a variable of concern for homeless adults residing in Tucson. Twenty-eight percent of the ASSET participants reported having chronic medical problems which require treatment. Although the ASSET project screens out adults with co-morbidity issues that require medication, 16% reported taking other prescribed medications regularly. Only 4% of the ASSET participants had been receiving medical disability pensions. When asked at intake whether they had experienced medical problems within the past month, 57% reported having no medical problems. Twenty-four percent reported having medical problems between 1 and 10 days, 12% reported having medical problems between 21 and 30 days, and 7% reported having medical problems between 11 and 20 days.

As three of the four ASSET treatment objectives included (1) reduction of alcohol and drug use, (2) increase in employment, and (3) increase in health status, questions regarding how much the participant was bothered by these issues and importance of treatment for these issues were analyzed. Forty-two percent and 41% reported being extremely bothered by their alcohol or drug problem respectively. Seventy-seven percent indicated that treatment was extremely important for their alcohol problem and 73% indicated that treatment was extremely important for their drug problem.

Those who reported being extremely bothered by their employment issues totaled 43%. Fifty-one percent reported that it was extremely important for them to get treatment regarding their employment problems.

Finally when questioned about their health status only 19% reported being extremely bothered by their health problems. However, 27% reported that it was extremely important for them to obtain treatment for their medical problems.

Implications for Practice, Research and Policy

Several implications for practice, research and policy are evidenced. First, as mentioned as a barrier to the ASSET project implementation, new projects must address the NIMBY Syndrome at least six months prior to funding approval. In fact, the NIMBY Syndrome should be addressed as an ongoing issue in one's city as six months is actually a very short time frame to address such a large issue. Several routes or methods to site acquisition should occur simultaneously.

Secondly, recruitment of participants through other referral agencies takes a great deal of time and energy. A recruitment/enrollment plan should be developed in advance with adequate staff time devoted to this task. Collaboration with counselors or case managers at referring agencies is critical if referrals are to occur on a regular basis.

A third implication for practice in a research demonstration project is that there must be frequent and ongoing communication between the clinical and research staff. Ideally several meetings/discussions between the two sets of staff should occur prior to enrolling clients into the project. Once the project is underway weekly meetings to address ongoing and new issues is recommended.

Finally, treatment service projects which include random assignment must address the random assignment issue with the clinical staff. How to tell potential clients about the alternatives that the random assignment provides must be specified and even written out in a script form for the clinical staff. Continuous discussion about why random assignment is important should occur. When preliminary research results are available, these reports should be presented to both the research and clinical staff in a discussion session. Allowing clinical staff to talk about the preliminary results empowers them as clinical researchers and includes them in the research component.

In summary, large research demonstration projects serving the adult homeless population can provide a wealth of information regarding the participants to be served, intervention effectiveness, and recommendations for future research and clinical issues. Only in examining what projects have provided in the past and how participants were or were not affected by their experience can the field move forward and become more effective in approach.

REFERENCES

Bissell, N. (1992). Background information on clients served at the Primavera Foundation Shelter for the Homeless. Unpublished report.

Black, M. (1992). El Rio Health Clinic Status of Records Report. Unpublished report.

Condelli, W.S. & Dunteman, G.H. (in press) Methodological issues to consider when predicting retention in the therapeutic community. (To be published in the National Institute of Drug Abuse Research Monograph on Therapeutic Community Treatment Research.)

DeLeon, G. (1988). Therapeutic community research facts: What we know. *Therapeutic Communities of America News*, Summer 1-2.

DeLeon, G. (1986). The Therapeutic Community for Substance Abuse: Perspective and Approach. *Therapeutic Communities for Addictions: Readings in Theory, Research and Practice*, G. DeLeon and J. Ziegenfuss, (Eds.). Springfield, IL.: Charles C Thomas.

Erickson, J.R., Estrada, A., and Stevens, S.J. (1992). Risk for AIDS among homeless intravenous drug users (IDUs) in Southern Arizona. Paper to be presented at the American Public Health Association, Washington, D.C.

Glider, P., Mullen, R., Davis, C. & Ker, M. (in review). Substance abuse treatment in a jail setting: A therapeutic community model.

McNamara, J. (1991). Clinical Records: Gateway LARC Detoxification Center, Unpublished Report.

Mullen, R. (1992). The Prison-Based Therapeutic Community. In *Introductory Training: The Teaching and Therapeutic Community for Drug Abusing Offenders*, N. Arbiter and R. Mullen, (Eds.). Tucson: Amity, Inc.

Rom-Rymer, J. (1981). An empirical assessment of Mowrer's theory of psychopathology applied to a therapeutic community. Doctoral dissertation, Florida State University, Ann Arbor, MI: University Microfilms International.

Simpson, D.D. and Sells, S.B. (1982). Effectiveness of treatment for drug abuse: An overview of the DARP research program. *Advances in Alcohol and Substance Abuse*, 2 (1), 7-29.

Stevens, S.J. and Glider, P. (in press). Therapeutic communities: Substance abuse treatment for women. To be published in the National Institute of Drug Abuse Research Monograph on Therapeutic Community Treatment Research.

Wexler, H.K., Falkin, P. and Lipton, D. (1990). Outcome evaluation of prison TC's for substance abuse treatment. *Criminal Justice and Behavior, 17*, 71-72.

Case Management and Supported Housing in Chicago: The Interaction of Program Resources and Client Characteristics

Michael R. Sosin, MSW, PhD
Joan Schwingen
Jane Yamaguchi, MSW

SUMMARY. The described program provides extended interventions for Chicago adults who abuse alcohol or drugs and also have homeless experience. This program responds to evidence that (1) members of the relevant population cannot easily access either long-term substance abuse treatment or programs that serve other individuals who are homeless, (2) individuals who are both homeless and have substance abuse problems tend to be poorly matched to the programs to which they have access, and (3) a cycle of substance abuse and homelessness occurs as the lack of stable material, residential, and social support inhibits the commitment to recovery. There are two sets of interventions: a case management plus supported housing option that provides individuals with apartments for up to eight months while providing many other types of support, and a case management only

Michael R. Sosin is Professor at The University of Chicago, The School of Social Service Administration, 969 East 60th Street, Chicago, IL 60637. Joan Schwingen is Associate Director at Travelers and Immigrants Aid of Chicago. Jane Yamaguchi is Research Assistant at The School of Social Service Administration, The University of Chicago.

[Haworth co-indexing entry note]: "Case Management and Supported Housing in Chicago: The Interaction of Program Resources and Client Characteristics." Sosin, Michael R., Joan Schwingen, and Jane Yamaguchi. Co-published simultaneously in the *Alcoholism Treatment Quarterly* (The Haworth Press, Inc.) Vol. 10, No. 3/4, 1993, pp. 35-50; and: *Treatment of the Chemically Dependent Homeless: Theory and Implementation in Fourteen American Projects* (ed: Kendon J. Conrad, Cheryl I. Hultman, and John S. Lyons) The Haworth Press, Inc., 1993, pp. 35-50. Multiple copies of this article/chapter may be purchased from The Haworth Document Delivery Center [1-800-3-HAWORTH: 9:00 a.m. - 5:00 p.m. (EST)].

35

option that provides help in locating residences along with the supports. Both use a "progressive independence" approach which begins by ameliorating immediate tangible needs and builds toward a collaborative relationship that focuses on other issues. Preliminary information suggests that the programs can be implemented in ways that deal with core client concerns and retain clients in treatment longer than is typical.

BACKGROUND

The economic environment of Chicago reflects the profound problems of the 1980s and 1990s. For example, even if the average income of the city was well above average, the unemployment rate stood at 11.3% at the time of the 1990 census. The median rent was a hefty $445 per month, while welfare benefits were set at only $367 for a family of three ($154 for one individual). Rigid rules currently reduce the utility of these inadequate income maintenance programs; the General Assistance program sanctioned one-quarter of the caseload in one six month period (Sosin et al., 1988). And family supports are in decay in this urban area, one of the five cities that account for a majority of a dramatic expansion in the concentration of poverty over the 1970s and perhaps beyond (Jargowsky and Bane, 1991).

Many Chicago adults, including those with substance abuse problems, seem to be at risk of homelessness when they have been unemployed for many years in this weak economy. The direct loss of the domicile primarily occurs when "vulnerable" individuals lack the very tangible resources that are becoming more difficult to maintain–income maintenance benefits, access to inexpensive housing, and access to relatives who house them (Sosin, 1992). But substance abuse complicates matters. It is a precondition for vulnerability; it directly predicts repeated or lengthy losses of the domicile; it increases the probability that non-economic factors also lead to homelessness. Indeed, certain types of "disaffiliation" from conventional society (Bahr and Caplow, 1974) and familiarity with unconventional life-styles are more common among individuals with substance abuse problems who are homeless than among those who are vulnerable but domiciled (Sosin and Bruni, forthcoming).

Adults who have homeless experience may also not benefit from substance abuse interventions. For example, they are too heavily involved in the struggle for material sustenance to place a high priority on recovery, are skeptical about the utility of intangible services, and have difficulty in accessing programs to which they might be attracted. Locally, while those agencies funded by the Illinois Department of Alcohol and Substance Abuse cater to financially needy individuals to such a degree that half of their clients have some experience with homelessness (Sosin et al., 1988), the programs are insufficient. Longer term halfway houses and inpatient treatment programs that provide at least a temporary domicile are rare, and these options also are unavailable to adults who cannot meet the demand to immediately pay part of the cost of care (Chicago Coalition for the Homeless, 1989). Few if any programs develop specific methods to combat the economic or social factors that lead to homelessness (and limit motivation to recover). Publicly supported outpatient programs also have high caseloads, tend to focus on clients who are mandated to attend, and rarely have the resources needed to make a special effort to attract or treat adults who are homeless. Long-term residential programs are generally organized under the expectation that clients become active members of a sober community that becomes a prime focus of their lives. Communal life does not appear to be attractive to individuals who desire economic advancement and do not easily attach to others; these facilities have been found to house older, more stable, and less disaffiliated men and thus to fail to serve men and women who typify the homeless population (Sosin et al., 1988).

More generally, adults who lack a domicile also fail to share the traits that seem prerequisite for the success of many apparently efficacious substance abuse interventions (Miller and Hester, 1986)—high social status, firm social supports, stable relations with family members, and secure employment (Bromet and Moos, 1977; Fischer and Breakey, 1987; Koegel and Burnham, 1987; Sosin et al., 1988). And few programs addressing homelessness attempt to restore economic stability, while many are wary of serving individuals who have substance abuse problems.

MODEL OF CARE

The Chicago "First Things First" project, a collaboration between researchers at the University of Chicago and service providers at Travelers and Immigrants Aid of Chicago, develops (and tests the value of) service models that compensate for factors that compromise interventions by focusing on residential instability and its causes as well as treatment for substance abuse. Because long term treatment options are particularly lacking, the project recruits individuals with homeless experience out of 30 day residential treatment programs (one for men, one for women, one for veterans). This is accomplished through periodic screening sessions that determine whether each cooperating participant in the 30 day programs meets the criteria for homelessness. Those who do, approximately forty percent of the residents, are basically randomly assigned to one of two treatment programs or to a control group.

The first column of Table 1, which reports characteristics of those who

Table 1

DESCRIPTIVE STATISTICS BY INTERVENTION GROUP

Characteristic	Total Sample [a] Statistic (SD) (n=145)	Housing Group Statistic (SD) (n=97)	Case Management Only Statistic (SD) (n=48)
GENDER			
% Female	35.9	41.2	25.0*
ETHNICITY			
% White	7.6	6.2	10.6
% African American	88.2	89.7	85.1
% Hispanic	3.5	4.2	2.1
% Other	0.7	0.0	2.1
MEAN AGE	34.2 (7.94)	34.4 (8.37)	33.9 (7.07)
MEAN YEARS OF EDUCATION	11.8 (1.82)	11.6 (1.99)	12.0 (1.40)
MEAN NUMBER OF MONTHS HOMELESS (lifetime)	28.9 (34.98)	30.0 (33.24)	26.6 (38.47)
% ADMITTING PROBLEM WITH ALCOHOL	78.4	79.1	77.1

38

% ADMITTING PROBLEM WITH DRUGS	81.3	76.9	89.6*
ADDICTION SEVERITY INDEX [b] AREA MEAN SCORES:			
ALCOHOL	0.43 (.30)	0.45 (0.30)	0.38 (0.30)
DRUG	0.23 (.15)	0.22 (0.15)	0.24 (0.15)
PSYCHOLOGICAL	0.34 (.19)	0.34 (0.19)	0.32 (0.19)
LEGAL	0.16 (20)	0.15 (0.19)	0.16 (0.22)
MEDICAL	0.25 (32)	0.25 (0.32)	0.26 (0.32)
SOCIAL SUPPORT	0.38 (20)	0.39 (0.19)	0.37 (0.22)
EMPLOYMENT	0.86 (.18)	0.88 (0.15)	0.81** (0.22)

For Housing v. Case Management Only differences

*p<.10

**p<.05

[a] Note: Size of n varies from 133 to 145 due to non-responses.

[b] In each treatment problem area, higher scores indicate greater severity (need for additional treatment).

McLellan, A.T., Luborsky, L., Woody, G., & O'Brien, C.P. (1980). An improved diagnostic evaluation instrument for substance abuse patients: The Addiction Severity Index. Journal of Nervous and Mental Disease, 168(1), 26-33.

actually enter the project programs, suggests that the recruited clients generally have alcohol problems, and that the majority also report drug problems. Clients tend to be low income, predominantly African American adults whose average age and level of education are typical for Chicagoans who lack a domicile. They have more than two years of homeless experience on average, and are more frequently male than female.

Treatment Alternatives

The two project treatments to which clients are recruited contrast with available care in that they assume, among other things, that individuals need to be attached to some type of stable or longer term housing before they can easily contemplate recovery and work toward financial independence. Admittedly, the most useful housing strategy remains in doubt. Some local experts assert that clients can obtain a domicile from otherwise reluctant landlords or loosely supervised housing situations if outside caseworkers agree to provide supports. But others are skeptical of this and suggest that individuals who have substance abuse problems and unstable residential histories may refuse services unless a domicile is directly provided. The project accordingly tests two options (clients are offered only one): (1) a Case Management and Supported Housing option, in which clients are provided residences along with a particular type of case management, and (2) a Case Management Only option, in which clients are provided case managers who help them look for private housing and also render the case management services. After six to eight months of intensive services, all individuals are eligible for six months of less intensive case management.

In contrast, those in the control group obtain usual care in the 30 day treatment setting, which often consists of referrals to outpatient programs, some basic help in applying for income maintenance benefits, and referrals to long-term inpatient programs. For reasons noted above, we estimate that less than fifteen percent enter long-term inpatient programs, and are not confident that other referrals are successful.

Housing

The aim of the housing intervention is to help clients learn to live independently in an environment filled with temptation, not to master functioning in a controlled setting. Further, it is meant to reduce the chance that disaffiliation reduces the efficacy of the intervention as some clients reject particularly intensive interpersonal demands (Susser et al., 1990). Therefore, the housing option attempts to balance the need to maintain control with some degree of freedom. Workers deliver services, but clients are provided regular apartments in one of three buildings that serve low income tenants. To avoid unreasonable financial demands while still realistically working toward client independence, sliding scale rent copayments are collected after two months and gradually increase.

CASE MANAGEMENT:
THE PROGRESSIVE INDEPENDENCE MODEL

In both interventions, comprehensive case management is used to meet the need for an array of services–treatment for substance abuse, access to tangible resources, provision of family supports, help overcoming disaffiliation, and the like. But the choice of techniques is complex. The value of the most widely specified and researched form of case management, "assertive community treatment," is unknown because this approach has largely been studied for adults with persistent mental illnesses (Test, 1991). Indeed, assertive community treatment might be inappropriate for individuals with substance abuse problems, who are likely to reject close control; it encourages workers to actively eschew concern about client "dependency" and to even help with common daily chores. The alleged tendency of some individuals who have substance abuse problems to use relationships to avoid confronting addiction also threatens the utility of an approach that relies on intimate interaction.

On the other hand, interventions should not completely focus on a therapeutic approach, or on a "brokering" approach that stresses coordination and referral (Willenbring et al., 1991). Potential clients may not be ready for (or, given findings in the literature, benefit from) intense treatment; their chronic abuse problems, uncertain work histories, and periodic failure to maintain housing suggest that they need some support despite their desire to be independent. And if literature from the mental health field can be generalized, such approaches are not likely to be particularly successful (Bond et al., 1988; Test, 1991).

Our case management approach thus has developed into what we call a "progressive independence" model. One aspect of the model, the interactive style, can best be described as an attempt to eventually create a delicate balance in which workers recommend courses of action to clients through negotiation and contracting, while clients pursue the strategies, face frustrations, and attempt to make corrections with the worker's help. To be sure, all programs individualize services according to the particular abilities of clients. However, a norm has developed by which collaboration is the pursued goal until it becomes apparent that a certain client needs a greater level of support or that an issue (such as the application process for SSI) causes unusual difficulties for most clients.

The approach also mandates a series of standards that help ensure that clients take the personal responsibility needed to control abuse–these have an additional function of limiting the extent to which clients "making the loop" (Wiseman, 1970) misuse the program. Clients must sign contracts that lay out ambitious expectations of maintaining abstinence, making a full commitment to long-term recovery, participating in AA and out-patient treatment as well as weekly support groups, attending individual counseling and recreational activities, complying with unscheduled drug tests, cooperating with efforts to develop income and a budget plan, and taking steps to locate permanent housing. Those who fail to conform and do not demonstrate improvement after renegotiation of the contract are removed from the housing unit. This essentially means that individuals are allowed one relapse into substance abuse, and are removed for the second (case management services continue). While this is controversial among project staff, clients can also be suspended from case management services for a second relapse or for a general failure to cooperate. They may be reinstated when they demonstrate a willingness to participate actively and to commit to another contract.

IMPLEMENTING THE MODEL OF CARE

Early Stages

There is no common daily schedule; the two treatment models allow clients considerable freedom to work, visit with families, set up other needed services, and carry out other tasks. Nevertheless, certain activities occur in a general sequence. Because the progressive independence model asserts that tangible needs must be confronted immediately (to build trust and provide clients sufficient stability to deal with substance abuse and conditions that lead to homelessness), one time only assistance with security deposits (direct voucher payments) and household goods are made available under controlled conditions as clients are settled. Early sessions in both options encourage clients to pursue eligibility for benefit programs or employment (attorneys are consulted, as needed), and workers later assure continued access to resources (for example, by negotiating with income maintenance staff when benefits are terminated, acting as money managers or representative payees).

Under the assumption that conditions interact, the substance abuse problem is also immediately confronted through the mandate that clients attend 90 AA and other outpatient meetings in the first 90 days of the program. AA groups, which vary widely in style and accessibility, are chosen by clients through a process of negotiation based on how "serious" the program is; how open it is to new entrants; and whether it separates clients from others with whom they shared drugs and alcohol in the past. The clients should be trying out ways of analyzing barriers to maintaining sobriety as they negotiate appropriate programs.

Intermediate Stages

A collaborative relationship should develop further after tangible needs are met, clients develop a stable base, and program credibility is firmly established. Opportunities to consider issues occur naturally as clients come into contact with their families and begin to consider employment or other tasks, and are faced with some of the same pressures that previously led to both substance abuse and homelessness.

Interventions often become complex. Group sessions provide support and offer a forum for solving various problems that are closely bound with homelessness. Practical skills also are developed with the help of referrals to job training and internal classes on obtaining employment. Tangible needs, family problems, referrals to health care, and links to other programs also are considered in individual sessions. Workers spend much time transporting clients, and believe that much useful advice is dispensed during such informal encounters.

A cognitive behavioral "relapse prevention" package is used within the weekly group sessions as an aid in helping clients consider new ways of responding to situations that hinder the maintenance of sobriety. Largely based on the work of Marlatt (1985), the prevention package helps clients recognize triggers–situations which might cause them to relapse or otherwise deteriorate. Clients are encouraged to learn to stop and think about possible ways of dealing with these situations, rehearse solutions, try the new solutions, report on their success, and refine such strategies. For example, one client identified the high risk situation of cashing a benefit check at currency exchanges where he faces drug dealers. With the help of a worker, he considered various courses of action, from rehearsing ways of refusing the drug dealers to cashing a check when accompanied by a friend. This client eventually concluded that neither he nor his friends could oppose a drug dealer, and the case manager went with the client to cash his check, in this one instance modifying the original expectation of independent action.

Final Stages

Clients are seen less frequently after receiving up to eight months of intensive services. The focus is on maintenance or prevention of new problems rather than intensive treatment. Successful clients are encouraged to return to group meetings and outings to help inspire others; their graduation from housing, in particular, is treated as an occasion for celebration and recognition of a milestone.

Workers help clients who complete the housing program look for permanent quarters near the eighth month limit (help varies from making telephone calls, to locating vacancies which the client must pursue, to canvassing neighborhoods), and will even help with the move. Eventually, clients in either option should locate permanent employment and housing and pursue longer term goals. For example, one 29 year old woman successfully completed the housing component, applied for a temporary holiday season job, and was eventually hired full time; she has been sober for over a year and is planning her wedding. One 37 year old male case management client signed his first apartment lease, obtained SSI, and is working toward obtaining a GED and employment.

Relapses

A perhaps expected difficulty is that clients seem to relapse at a considerable rate–even if both clients and workers believe that drug screens, recontracting after relapses, and eviction of clients from housing after two relapses helps maintain sobriety. As might be predicted, workers believe that some of the more vulnerable clients are those who isolate themselves in their apartments or those who proceed from grandiose expectations that they will immediately improve to withdrawal upon failure.

Another first impression is that challenges that lead to relapse occur as clients continue to rely on family and friends for support or even material help, even though a small proportion of relatives and perhaps half of the friends of clients abuse substances (according to replies to questionnaire items). Given their tendency to fully identify with social networks, clients have particular problems refusing offered substances that are part of the network culture. For women, additional concerns center on the need to prove sobriety to regain legal custody of children, many of whom are housed by relatives who do not understand that clients must remove themselves from family activities where drink or drugs are available. Finally, some workers wonder whether outpatient programs (or housing programs used by case management clients) so fully teach clients to identify with their peer group in treatment that they inhibit development of the sophisticated skills needed to interact with, but remain wary of, members of the long-standing social network. Workers summarize this by suggesting that they must negotiate not only material needs, but also cultural "worlds."

One helpful elaboration of the intervention occurred because clients also have come to refer to the "old world," which included the traps of drug and alcohol use, and their "new world." It has become possible to use changes in health (a "healthy look"), physical appearance, and behavior (such as a new unwillingness to trade popular athletic shoes for drugs) to reinforce continuance of the new. The new apparently has become valued–partly due to the tangible goods the program provides–and this seems to help clients focus their strategies for refusing offers to return to drug or alcohol use. Given the dearth of social opportunities for poor adults who wish to avoid alcohol and drugs, the program also has become involved in arranging picnics and outings that help reinforce that enjoyment can be achieved along with abstinence.

Increasingly, clients identify relationship problems that are precipitants of substance abuse and that also may be linked to homelessness. In the groups, clients prefer to use behavioral strategies to deal with these rather than the perception-oriented approaches that seem to be stressed more by Marlatt. Common strategies include reducing lengths of visits, limiting topics of discussion, leaving when certain topics or tensions arise, as well as "self talk" strategies to improve their own sense of efficacy even when others tell them otherwise.

IMPLEMENTATION ADJUSTMENTS

Housing

It proved possible to obtain twenty unit blocks of rooms at three recently renovated apartment buildings, under the condition that the program paid the rent. Perhaps arrangements were readily concluded because building managers appreciated guaranteed rents; poor clients have difficulty in meeting monthly payments in the local economy. Our lack of problems with the community may be due to the low profile of the program, its location within buildings already renting to low income individuals, and its reliance on an approach that stresses the conventional residential nature of offered dwellings.

However, management of the buildings objected when some clients became inebriated, brought in "undesirable" friends, or failed to maintain a reasonable level of sanitation. While attempting to maintain a balance of restrictions and freedom, staff members have had to assume increasing control over the residences, even at times providing detailed guidance with such tasks as upkeep of the apartment. Regular meetings between workers and managers have been established to discuss such issues as who has responsibility for responding to noisy parties (the resident manager attempts this first), or who informs clients that their behavior threatens to demand eviction (this is left to the case manager). One full-time resource developer now deals with physical maintenance of housing.

For clients who were not in the housing program, appropriate residences were difficult to find; help with security deposits is insufficient if the rent is too high. Interim arrangements often were made with halfway houses or long-term residential programs. The research will eventually assess if clients can remain in the programs when provided supports of a case manager. Interestingly, clients generally preferred to make their own arrangements and double up with relatives or mates rather than accept such commonly available alternatives as shelters or transitional housing programs.

Client Recruitment

Recruitment of clients to the housing option seems to be straightforward because 78 percent of approached clients accept the offer. However, only thirty percent of the approached clients participate in the case management only option–which, to be sure, is comparable or superior to other reported participation rates (Stark, 1992; Baekeland and Lundwall, 1975). One difficulty arose because staff at the 30 day programs referred exiting clients to outpatient programs where they were counseled by someone called a "case manager." Given the ambiguity of the term, staff at first sometimes viewed our services as superfluous. But our case managers, who were aware of the need to build relations within the organizational setting (Willenbring et al., 1991), improved cooperation by providing information about the flexible types of offered supports, including tangible goods, help in locating housing, and encouragement for clients to continue outpatient treatment.

Case managers also have felt the need to be quite active in explaining the program to clients who are still in the thirty day programs. A formal orientation describes and presents written explanations of services, gives examples of client newsletters and other benefits, and even provides clients with a transportation token to attend the next meeting. Workers speculate that participation in the case management only option is more likely when clients receive needed help with transportation, desire to be involved in groups with housing clients they know, and are interested in the offered recreational activities.

PRELIMINARY STATISTICAL ANALYSES

Table 1 also compares clients interviewed by March 30, 1992 who have accepted each option (control clients are not analyzed for this paper). Even if a much more limited proportion of clients accepted the case management only package, results uncover no statistically significant differences in alcohol or drug symptomatology, age, education, psychological problems, and experience with homelessness. Case management only clients have slightly fewer employment problems and, using the .10 level of significance, are more likely to admit to a drug problem. Again using the .10 significance level, women are somewhat less common among case management only clients. Perhaps they perceive less need because they often can return to a "doubled up" situation with relatives or obtain AFDC.

Figure 1, which compares the length of stay of clients while taking into account that many individuals are still in the programs, summarizes calculations that suggest that close to half (42 percent) remain in the case management only option for at least three months, while about three-quarters (78 percent) remain in the housing option for this length of time.

FIGURE 1. Cumulative Survival Rates–Housing vs. Case Management

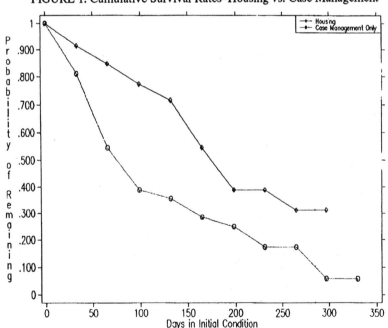

About half (48 percent) remain in housing for six months; the rate of leaving seems to increase over time. These rates of retention are certainly far from ideal, but a tentative conclusion is that both options are successful in relative terms; research (generally not focusing on adults who have homeless experience) suggests that at least half of clients treated for alcohol problems in typical outpatient programs drop out by the fourth session, eighty percent drop out within the first three months, and less than twenty percent of those treated in residential programs continue for at least three months (Stark, 1992; Baekeland and Lundwall, 1975). The comparative advantages of the housing program also seem clear, because the above data do not take into account the continuation in case management of clients removed from the provided dwelling.

There is some relation between client traits at entry and length of stay in the program as determined by "survival analyses" (Allison, 1984).[1] To be sure, given that the sample is small and many clients have been in the program for a short period, the .10 level of significance is used and the analyses must be considered exploratory. But the preliminary results suggest that, for both the housing clients and case management clients, the rate of retention is lower for clients with greater previous homeless experience. The housing program, in which clients interact more with each other, less fully retains individuals who say they lacked friends as a child; the case management program, in which clients interact more with workers, less fully retains those who believe they did not have close childhood relationships with significant adults. Individuals who report having greater drug problems also are retained at lower rates in the housing program, while those with greater alcohol problems are retained at lower rates in the case management program. Whatever the specific findings, the analyses provide evidence that some types of clients benefit more from each option.

Further analyses suggest that measures of the number of relatives and friends in the social network who abuse substances also affect the retention rates. Most such relations nevertheless are not sustained when the individual's own previous level of abuse is included, which suggests that the severity of personal substance abuse is a major cause of the relation of outcomes to the nature of the network chosen before coming into contact with the program (data on the current network is being collected). However, those whose friends abuse drugs remain in the case management condition for shorter periods even with levels of personal substance abuse held constant. The relation is only rendered insignificant (neither variable retains significance) when previous legal problems are also controlled. Apparently, previously having friends who abuse drugs, and personal involvement in criminal conduct, represent a set of conditions that make continuation in this option less attractive.

CONCLUSION

Compared to other programs–which admittedly do not focus on adults who have homeless experience–both treatment conditions seem to retain clients at above average rates. The provision of housing is, to be sure, more powerful in that it approximately doubles the rate of accepting services and the time spent in care. Perhaps the need is so great that housing is a strong incentive, or perhaps other clients are unable to emphasize recovery when they have concerns about housing. Nevertheless, there are sufficient differences in background traits of those who accept each option, and in traits of those who continue longer, to suspect that the programs might best target somewhat different individuals.

More generally, the progressive independence model seems to show some promise in the sense that the emphasis on tangible needs may help retain clients in both options. Perhaps this model should continue to evolve in ways that consider relations with referral programs, balance independent living with the practical and relationship problems clients demonstrate, and attempt to retain those who are isolated or are particularly chronic in homelessness or levels of substance abuse.

NOTE

1. The models "censor" individuals who are still in programs at the current length of stay. They also censor housing program completers at the point they graduate, because they might stay longer if allowed by the program. Both equations use Weibull models.

REFERENCES

Allison, P.D. (1984). *Event history analysis: Regression for longitudinal data.* Beverly Hills: Sage Publications.

Baekeland, F. & Lundwall, L. (1975). Dropping out of treatment: A critical review. *Psychological Bulletin, 82*(5), 738-783.

Bahr, H. & Caplow, T. (1974). *Old men: Drunk and sober.* NY: New York University Press.

Bond, G., Miller, L., Krumwied R., & Ward, R. (1988). Assertive case management in three CMHCs: A controlled study. *Hospital and Community Psychiatry, 39*(4), 411-418.

Bromet, E.J. & Moos, R. (1977). Environmental resources and the post-treatment functioning of alcoholic patients. *Journal of Health and Social Behavior, 18*, 326-335.

Chicago Coalition for the Homeless. (1989). *Findings of the task force on alcoholism and other drug abuse services.* Chicago, IL.: Author.

Fischer, P.J. & Breakey, W.J. (1987). Profile of the Baltimore homeless with alcohol problems. *Alcohol and Research World, 11*(3), 36-37.

Jargowsky, P.A. & Bane, M.J. (1991). Ghetto poverty in the United States, 1970-1980. In C. Jencks, & P. Peterson (Eds.), *The urban underclass* (pp. 235-273). Washington, D.C.: The Brookings Institution.

Koegel, P. & Burnam, M.A. (1987). Traditional and non-traditional homeless alcoholics. *Alcohol and Research World, 11*(3), 28-33.

Marlatt, G.A. (1985). Part I: Relapse prevention: General overview. In G.A. Marlatt & J.R. Gordon (Eds.), *Relapse prevention: Maintenance strategies in the treatment of addictive behaviors* (pp. 3-348). New York: Guilford Press.

Miller W.R. & Hester, R.K. (1986). The Effectiveness of alcoholism treatment: What research reveals. In W.R. Miller & N. Heather (Eds.), *Treating addictive behaviors: Processes of change* (pp. 121-174). New York: Plenum Press.

Sosin, M. (1992). Homeless and vulnerable meal program users: A comparison study. *Social Problems, 39*(2), 170-88.

Sosin, M., Colson, P., & Grossman, S. (1988). *Homelessness in Chicago: Poverty and pathology, social institutions and social change.* Chicago: Chicago Community Trust and School of Social Service Administration, University of Chicago.

Sosin, M. & Bruni, M. (forthcoming). Homelessness and alcoholism.

Stark, M.J. (1992). Dropping out of substance abuse treatment: A clinically oriented review. *Clinical Psychology Review, 12*, 93-116.

Susser, E., Goldfinger, S. M., & White, A. (1990). Some clinical approaches to the homeless mentally ill. *Community Mental Health Journal, 26*(5), 463-480.

Test, M.A. (1991). The Training in Community Living model: Delivering treatment and rehabilitation services through a continuous treatment team. In R. P. Liberman (Ed.), *Handbook of Psychiatric Rehabilitation,* New York: Pergamon Press.

Wiseman, J.P. (1970). *Stations of the lost.* Englewood Cliffs, NJ: Prentice-Hall.

Willenbring, M. L., Ridgely, M. S., Stinchfield, R., & Rose, M. (1991). *Application of case management in alcohol and drug dependence: Matching techniques and populations* (DHHS Pub. No. ADM 91-1766) Rockville, MD: U.S. Department of Health and Human Services, Public Health Service, and ADAMHA.

POLITICS AND PROGRAMS: NEW ORLEANS, NEWARK, NEW HAVEN

The New Orleans Homeless Substance Abusers Program

James D. Wright, PhD
Joel A. Devine, PhD
Neil Eddington, PhD

SUMMARY. In New Orleans, the United States' 25th largest city, the problems of substance abuse and homelessness are exacerbated by some unique economic and cultural characteristics of the city. This article describes the development of a program designed to achieve sobriety, residential stability, economic independence, and family re-integration within this context. The theory and philosophy behind this program are presented and the political, administrative, and clinical barriers to implementation are described. Baseline data from the initial 670 clients served are presented, and early findings are discussed.

James D. Wright and Joel A. Devine are affiliated with the Department of Sociology, Tulane University. Neil Eddington is affiliated with the Center for Supervised Residential Services.

[Haworth co-indexing entry note]: "The New Orleans Homeless Substance Abusers Program." Wright, James D., Joel A. Devine, and Neil Eddington. Co-published simultaneously in the *Alcoholism Treatment Quarterly* (The Haworth Press, Inc.) Vol. 10, No. 3/4, 1993, pp. 51-64; and: *Treatment of the Chemically Dependent Homeless: Theory and Implementation in Fourteen American Projects* (ed: Kendon J. Conrad, Cheryl I. Hultman, and John S. Lyons) The Haworth Press, Inc., 1993, pp. 51-64. Multiple copies of this article/chapter may be purchased from The Haworth Document Delivery Center [1-800-3-HAWORTH: 9:00 a.m. - 5:00 p.m. (EST)].

51

INTRODUCTION

The New Orleans Homeless Substance Abusers Program (NOHSAP) is an NIAAA-funded, residentially based, adult resocialization demonstration project targeted to homeless alcoholics and drug abusers in the Greater New Orleans area. With a city population of about half a million and a metropolitan area population of approximately 1.3 million, New Orleans is the nation's twenty-fifth largest city. The city ranks third in its overall poverty rate and in the rate of child poverty (see U.S. Bureau of the Census, 1985; Children's Defense Fund, 1992); poverty in the city is heavily concentrated within the 70% black majority. Estimates of the size of the city's one-night homeless population vary from 5,000 to 12,000, of whom about 80% are African-Americans and about 25% are women.

The rate of alcohol abuse among the nation's homeless is reliably estimated to exceed 40%; among homeless men, it is close to 50% (Wright, 1989a, 1989b). (The true rate of alcohol abuse among the US population as a whole is not known to any degree of precision; most experts in the field use a "rule of thumb" figure of about 10 percent [Fisk, 1984; Institute of Medicine, 1988, p. 60]. Assuming this to be an indicative value, alcohol abuse is therefore some four times more widespread among the homeless than among the domiciled population.) In addition, some 15-20% of the homeless also abuse drugs other than alcohol. Thus, alcohol and drug abuse are arguably the most common health problems associated with homelessness, probably surpassing even mental illness in extent. "In whatever setting homeless adults are studied, alcoholism is the most frequent single disorder diagnosed" (Institute of Medicine, 1988, p. 60).

Alcohol and drug problems are understandably more common among the homeless of New Orleans than among homeless populations in other cities. The city's attitude about alcohol use is aptly expressed in its world-renowned motto, "Laissez les bon temps rouler" ("Let the good times roll"). Many cities tolerate public drunkenness; life in New Orleans frequently demands it. Bars are open 24 hours a day; beer, wine, and even hard liquor can be purchased in every convenience store. There are even drive-through frozen daiquiri shops in the city. Also, as the nation's largest port and the port nearest to South America, the city is a principal point of entry for narcotics and so the crack epidemic is every bit as harsh in New Orleans as in other major cities. In consequence, the New Orleans Task Force on Hunger and Homelessness has estimated that three-quarters of the city's homeless abuse alcohol, and that more than half abuse other drugs.

Except for the small programs for homeless veterans operated through the Center for Supervised Residential Services, a seven-day detoxification program now run through the Salvation Army, and a traditional residential treatment program for recovering substance abusers called Bridge House (total capacity of about 50), services for homeless or indigent substance abusers such as transitional housing, counseling, rehabilitation, aftercare, or extended treatment simply do not exist. As the nation's third poorest city, New Orleans offers very little in the area of social and human services, least of all to the homeless.

TREATMENT GOALS AND INTERVENTION PHILOSOPHY

NOHSAP is designed to achieve four principal goals: (1) an alcohol and drug free existence (permanent sobriety); (2) residential stability (permanent housing of more than minimal adequacy); (3) economic independence (jobs and incomes adequate to sustain an independent existence); and (4) a reduction in family estrangement. Our hope has been to demonstrate that with proper, well-designed interventions, even homeless addicts can be successfully reintegrated into the larger society and become productive, functioning, independent adults.

The general philosophy behind the NOHSAP intervention–and indeed behind all residential treatment programs–is that one cannot begin to address the alcohol and drug problems of homeless substance abusers until they are first stabilized residentially, that is, until they are provided with a clean, secure, and comfortable place to live. We therefore follow the prevailing opinion among alcohol and drug professionals that the key to successful treatment is to provide social and physical environments where sobriety is positively valued (Korenbaum and Burney, 1987). This, needless to say, is not the environment one encounters on the streets. Indeed, even acknowledging that many people are homeless precisely because of a pattern of chronic alcohol and drug abuse, it is worth emphasizing that drunkenness provides many positive benefits for a homeless person, and that high rates of alcohol and drug abuse will continue to prevail among the homeless so long as this remains true. Thus, the NOHSAP services package is specifically designed to provide a residential environment where sobriety is the norm and where independent living is positively encouraged.

We also believe that sobriety, like drunkenness, is best conceptualized as *learned* behavior and thus requires practice; therefore, we consider relapse to be an inherent and unavoidable aspect of recovery (Brown, 1985; Miller et al., 1982). Through episodes of sobriety and relapse, the recovering abuser practices and then masters a substance-free life-style. One must first *unlearn* the dysfunctional behaviors of the past and then learn (or in many cases, *relearn*) more functional patterns of behavior for the present and future. The essence of our intervention is to provide the proper unlearning and learning (resocialization) environment and to create a social and physical context that rewards and encourages these changes within the substance-abusive self. Periods of relapse, while certainly not encouraged, are generally tolerated; treatment is not denied or halted when persons exhibit the patterns of behavior that caused them to need treatment in the first place.

Chronic alcohol and drug use often serves a range of positive functions for a homeless individual (e.g., it dulls physical and emotional pain, induces euphoria, offers sociability, fills idle time). Treatment programs that attempt to address the alcohol or drug issue without also addressing the more basic problems for which alcohol or drug abuse is the client's solution are doomed or, at best, ineffectual. To emphasize, homeless people have many good reasons for getting and staying drunk. NOHSAP tries to provide good reasons for them to get and stay sober.

As we discuss later, the patterns of co-occurrence among alcohol abuse, drug abuse and mental and physical illness are strong ones, and there is consequently little doubt that the alcohol and drug abusers are, in general, the most seriously disabled subgroup within the homeless population. This is also the subgroup for whom employment or permanent long-term housing has traditionally been the least likely. It is all too easy to assume that these multiple disabilities are inherent to the homeless substance abuser and are therefore largely intractable. On the other hand, it may well be that appropriate systems of intervention and care have never been offered or assessed. NOHSAP is, in its very essence, an experiment to test the proposition that there is hope even for the most debilitated and problematic among the homeless population.

INTERVENTION MODEL

NOHSAP is designed as a three-phase intervention: detoxification, transitional care, and extended care/independent living. Detox is a seven-day program of sobering up, initial introduction to AA and NA principles, twice-daily group meetings, some counselling, and limited assessment and case management.

Both individual and family detox facilities are available, though only the latter is provided through NOHSAP itself. The former operates via a sub-contract between the State of Louisiana and the Center For Supervised Residential Services (CSRS), NOHSAP's clinical sub-contractor. Together, the two detox facilities have a seventeen unit, forty-bed capacity and a utilization rate approximating 100%. Access to social detoxification comes via referral from Charity Hospital, the local state-maintained hospital for the indigent located in downtown New Orleans. Referrals to family detox come from a variety of local facilities and organizations. Typically, there is a waiting list for social detoxification.

All clients are given an apartment. Single individuals have one to three roommates depending on whether the particular apartment has one or two bedrooms. Assignment is determined on a bed-available basis. Women with children are given their own apartment. All clients are responsible for cooking their own meals and keeping their apartments neat and clean. At the end of seven days, the vast majority of clients (the "controls") are transported back to Charity Hospital and discharged with a referral to one of the New Orleans Substance Abuse Clinics (NOSAC), a series of state-maintained out-patient facilities.

Transitional Care follows detoxification and is a twelve bed, twenty-one day program involving more extensive assessment, greater case management, twice-daily group meetings, placement in an off-campus alcohol or drug group, and general reinforcement of any positive steps taken during detox. Getting people to stop using drugs and alcohol proves to be the easy part of treatment; the hard part is teaching our clients how to deal with their sobriety. Much of the counselling in Transitional Care focusses on strategies for managing stress without alcohol or drugs. Many of our newly detoxed clients have no idea what to do with their free time, so we also do leisure time and recreational therapy. Many of our mothers have severely degraded parenting skills and so we provide parenting instruction as well.

Client placement in Transitional Care is determined via randomization out of a pool of detoxed clients whom the clinical staff has deemed eligible and appropriate for further placement. In cases where a client can be referred to an alternative in-patient transitional program, the external placement is made. However, this is a rare option. Space in Transitional Care is, of course, quite limited. Therefore, the pool of eligibles usually exceeds our placement capacity.

Similarly, clients who successfully complete the Transitional Care program become eligible for our twenty-bed Extended Care/Independent Living program. Extended Care is a twelve-month program and continues all the interventions and strategies begun during Transitional Care, except that we also add GED services, job training, and job placement. Clients live in the facility for free. All the mothers with children in the facility, whether in detox, transition, or extended care, must also volunteer four hours a week in our child care facility.

NOHSAP is sited in a forty-two unit apartment building in a pleasant residential section of New Orleans East. These are modern, newly-renovated apartments with the usual appliances, carpeting, central air conditioning, etc. In nearly all cases, these apartments are, overwhelmingly, the nicest places our clients have ever lived. Social detox is physically isolated from the rest of the campus by a fence; otherwise, clients mingle freely among themselves and with treatment staff. Administrative and research offices are mixed in among clients' apartments; the grounds are fenced in and provide ample opportunities for outdoor socializing (and for the children in the facility, play). The facility is bounded on its back side by a pretty bayou where clients occasionally fish. In all, the physical facility is a clean and peaceful sanctuary far removed (both physically and psychologically) from the grit and hard edge of life in the inner city from which our clients come.

NOHSAP saw its first clients in February 1991; to date, more than 700 clients have passed through the facility. Of these, about 500 are "control" clients who received seven days of detoxification and were then released back to the community and the remainder are "treatment" clients who were exposed to some period of Transitional or Transitional plus Extended Care. Outcome data are just now becoming available and so the successes of the program, if any, remain to be documented; still, it is already apparent that the relapse rate for our treatment clients is much lower than among controls, among whom more than 80% relapse within the first three months.

PROGRAM IMPLEMENTATION

The implementation of NOHSAP evolved into an interesting case study in the urban politics of NIMBYism, cronyism, race, and turf, one that eventually involved the city councils and mayors of two municipalities, hostile neighborhood associations, charges of plagiarism, forgery, and racism, inaccurate and hostile news stories in the local media–in short, all the "booming, buzzing confusion" of the urban political process.

Creating a residential treatment program for homeless addicts seems like a fine idea so long as the program is not placed in anyone's back yard. An ideal site in an outlying community was abandoned the day after the existence of the program was announced in the local paper because the police chief and city council saw absolutely no benefit whatever in bringing homeless addicts from the inner city into their community. Tensions between the city of New Orleans and its outlying suburbs, all of which are independent political entities, are historically deep; NOHSAP was seen as just another effort by the city to dump its problems on the suburbs. There were also efforts by developers, real estate people, community politicians, and neighborhood associations to prevent the facility's being placed anywhere *in* New Orleans as well; for a while, the Mayor of New Orleans and his War on Drugs officers were also opposed to the program's being sited anywhere in the city. The eventual site in New Orleans East was only chosen after a many-weeks-long process of meetings, deals, and conciliation.

NOHSAP's troubles with City Hall derived ultimately from the fact that some researchers from Tulane University had managed to raise about $3 million for an alcohol and drug intervention without the direct assistance of the Mayor's Office or his War on Drugs Office. People within the War on Drugs Office whose jobs were to raise alcohol and drug money for the city were especially incensed by this development and went so far as to claim publicly that the proposal had been plagiarized from work they had done. It was also suggested at one point that the Mayor's signature had been forged onto the letter of support that accompanied the original proposal submission and that the entire program was "just another bunch of white honkies wanting to do experiments on black people." That there was no truth to any of these allegations eventually stemmed the tide, but only after a private meeting between the Mayor of New Orleans and the President of Tulane University and lengthy negotiations with members of the City Council.

The political situation, tense to begin with, was inflamed still further by local media coverage. The existence of the program was announced in a lead story in the Metro Section of the New Orleans *The Times-Picayune* for Saturday, 6 October 1990, with the headline, "Homeless Addicts Get $3.1 Million." The article seemed intentionally inflammatory and managed to create the impression that the program was going to round up two or three thousand drug addicts from the streets of New Orleans, drop them off in the middle of the suburbs, and see how many of them would be able to make it back. While the later coverage was more positive, this initial story proved to be a total disaster whose repercussions were felt for several subsequent months.

Despite these political problems early on, an acceptable program site was eventually chosen. At the time the deal for the building was struck, it was run-down, largely abandoned, and a focus for drug activity in the neighborhood. (During the initial clean-up of the site, drug paraphernalia was swept from nearly every apartment.) The three-year guaranteed-occupancy lease made it possible for the landlord to undertake major renovations that spurred "clean up, paint up, fix up" efforts in adjacent complexes as well, and now, a year and a half later, it is obvious that NOHSAP has had a salutary effect on the whole neighborhood. As one New Orleans East apartment owner put it, we changed the clientele in the building from "poor, black and drunk" to "poor, black and sober" and with the benefit of hindsight nearly everyone would now admit that this was a stunning improvement. The complete absence of any incidents or security problems involving NOHSAP clients in the year and a half that we have occupied the site has certainly eased the anxieties of those living nearby.

TREATMENT ISSUES

Many barriers to adequate treatment of homeless substance abusers have been identified in the literature. One of the most important is the co-occurrence of psychiatric disorders. The rate of psychiatric disorder is significantly higher among homeless substance abusers than among the homeless in general (Wright, 1989b). Sadly, many mental health facilities refuse treatment to alcoholics or drug addicts, especially if they are still using, on the reasonable grounds that they are not equipped to provide alcohol or drug detoxification and rehabilitation services. Likewise, many alcohol and drug treatment facilities will refuse treatment to those who are also mentally ill, on largely the same grounds. What to do with homeless clients who are both alcohol-abusive or drug-abusive *and* mentally ill has therefore been extremely problematic. One strength of the NOHSAP services package is that mental health services as well as drug and alcohol treatment are essential program components, with both group and one-on-one therapy sessions offered to clients with these particular needs.

A second major treatment issue is the general lack of appropriate aftercare and long-term rehabilitative services. Most existing programs available to homeless substance abusers consist of short-term detoxification coupled (perhaps) with some counselling or rehabilitation, followed by release back to the streets, which is to say, release to exactly the environment that stimulated or exacerbated their substance abuse in the first place. Thus, many homeless substance abusers have been detoxified and "rehabilitated" dozens and dozens of times, almost always at considerable expense and with very inconsiderable success (Wright, 1989a). As we indicated above, detox followed by release to the streets represents NOHSAP's control condition and relapse runs to about 80% even in the first three months (this even though we provide an aftercare program for our detox-only clients).

Other key treatment issues that have been confronted during the first year include the following. First, virtually all our clients prove to be poly-substance abusive (or as we sometimes put it, "garbage can addicts"); we rarely encounter a "pure" alcoholic or a "pure" crack addict. To date, most clients have presented with at least an alcohol problem and a cocaine addiction; some will also do heroin when available, or psychedelics, or anything else the dealers have in the bag to offer.

Many of our clients freely admit to their cocaine addiction but deny that they have any problem with alcohol. Their attitude seems to be that alcohol is cheap, legal, and readily available (especially in New Orleans), its use is socially sanctioned, even encouraged (especially in New Orleans), and everyone drinks alcohol anyway (especially in New Orleans). So what's the problem? The problem, of course, is that most crack addicts use large quantities of alcohol to come down off the crack high or to sustain them between crack highs, and as a matter of fact, probably 90% of the relapse from cocaine addiction is first to alcohol and then back to cocaine and other drugs. Thus, one treatment issue lies in convincing our clients that the habitual and irresponsible use of alcohol is every bit as deleterious to their physical, social, and economic well-being as their habitual and irresponsible use of crack.

In addition to their homelessness and substance abuse, our clients have many additional problems that confound our efforts at treatment. In general, they are among the poorest of the poor and so they have very few resources that might sustain them through a period of recovery. Most of these addicts spend all their money on drugs and booze and so their nutritional status is very poor. Also, there are few if any groups in this society who smoke as many cigarettes as homeless substance abusive people. Many of the women avoid AFDC because they fear their children will be taken away if their circumstances become known; absent AFDC, of course, they are not eligible for Medicaid and therefore do not see a doctor when they need to. As for the men, in Louisiana only AFDC and SSDI recipients receive Medicaid, so their health problems are even worse. Nearly all our clients are deeply estranged from family, friend, and kin networks and therefore lack the social support necessary to "stay the course" of recovery.

Most clients who have been placed in Transitional Care remain for the full 21 days, but about half the clients placed in the Extended Care program have chosen to leave before completing the program. The exact reason for this pattern us unclear; our suspicion is that staying clean and sober for a month is within the capacity of most homeless addicts, but that the prospect of a full year of sobriety is more than a little daunting to many.

Many impoverished central city crack-addicted women, and thus many of our female clients, support their addiction via prostitution. Yet another treatment complication is thus the widespread incidence of venereal disorders, HIV positivity, and active AIDS infection. While on the point, it is worth mentioning that the incidence of the major classic venereal diseases–gonorrhea, syphilis, and chancroid–has declined sharply in most of the advanced industrial societies but has been increasing at epidemic rates among urban minority populations in the U.S. Recent studies in urban areas have found that the transmission of gonorrhea, syphilis, chancroid and HIV infections has been closely associated with the exchange of sex for drugs (Aral and Holmes, 1991). Women, particularly adolescent women, sometimes engage in very large numbers of sexual contacts to support their addiction.

Addicts are skillful manipulators with well-honed street survival skills. One particular challenge for treatment is to crack the toughened exterior to expose the powerless and needy individual inside. Virtually all our alcohol and drug counsellors are themselves former addicts and so they know every trick in the book, but they get taken in from time to time nonetheless. The women are particularly clever manipulators; many will try to use their children to curry special favors or attention.

Because poor women in New Orleans tend to have large numbers of children, we have at any one time as many as 30 children resident in our treatment facility. Like their mothers, they too pose special challenges. We have only recently begun an assessment program for the children; frankly, we were not prepared for the number of children we find ourselves dealing with and so our children's programming was a late addition to the services package. Still, it is obvious that many of our children suffer the congenital deficits resulting from their mothers' addictions; many are withdrawn and hostile when they first come to the program; many present with social and cognitive deficits that will haunt them throughout their lives. On entry, their nutritional and general health status is poor, many have not been properly immunized and dental problems are common. Still, in the face of it all, they are still children first and foremost; they want the things that all children want, romp and play the way all children play, respond to the same things that all children respond to. Given all the miseries they have suffered, they prove remarkably resilient and good-natured. And many respond in dramatically positive ways to the secure, stable residential environment that we provide them.

Some have questioned the wisdom of mixing our client populations as we do. Men, women, and children live together in adjacent apartments, socialize together, and in general, share their lives. We find that having lots of children around keeps the adults from acting out as much; it keeps people on their best behavior. Our treatment goal is independent living "out there" in the real world; our treatment facility attempts to model that world as closely as possible.

CLIENT CHARACTERISTICS AND TREATMENT OUTCOMES

Social and demographic correlates of alcohol and drug abuse among the homeless have also been rather extensively researched. A particularly detailed contribution is the Roth and Bean (1985) study of homeless persons in Ohio. Problem drinkers in their sample differed in many respects from the others. Demographically, they were disproportionally male, white, and old. As would be expected, they also had troubled marital histories (more likely than the remainder to be divorced or separated), more run-ins with the law, and higher rates of psychiatric impairment. They tended also to have been homeless and to have been unemployed for longer periods than the remainder of the sample, were more transient, and were more socially isolated. Finally, by self-report, they also showed higher levels of physical ill health (see Wright, 1989b, for clinical data on this last point). These data support the image of the homeless alcohol abuser as multiply disadvantaged and as exhibiting disproportionally high rates of poor physical, mental, and social health. Many other recent studies have reported essentially similar results (Koegel and Burnham, 1987; Fisher and Breakey, 1987; Ropers and Boyer, 1987; Wright, 1989b).

For the most part, our clients mirror the traits summarized above, with the exception that they are overwhelmingly African-American (82.2%). Our clients are relatively young, black men; the average age is in the lower 30s. About a third of the men are veterans. Most have some work history and a few job skills, but as a whole our clients are ill-prepared for employment in the post-industrial economy. Educational backgrounds are, of course, very limited, though more than half of the clients have had at least twelve years of education (see Table 1). About 90% of our clients were born and raised in Louisiana.

As per Table 1, additional baseline data from the 670 NOHSAP clients indicates that less than 40% have had previous episodes of homelessness. Just over half (52.5%) of the client population are multiple substance abusers; slightly less than half (47.6%) report an alcohol problem, while better than four-fifths (84.9%) abuse crack. While only about a quarter (26.9%) of the NOHSAP clients previously have undergone alcohol treatment, more than half (54.0%) have had prior non-alcohol drug treatment.

Client flow information is recorded in Diagram 1. Of the 670 NOHSAP clients, 57 have completed transitional care and entered the extended care/independent living program (ECIL). To date, ten clients have graduated ECIL and another 13 currently remain in the program. An additional 108 clients entered transitional care with all but seven completing the three-week program. The remaining 505 clients are controls. Following seven days of detox (see above, p. 5), controls typically are released back to the streets.

TABLE 1. – SELECTED DEMOGRAPHIC CHARACTERISTICS OF NOHSAP CLIENTS
(N = 670)

	#	%		#	%
RACE			AGE (years)		
African-American	551	82.2	19 – 24	65	9.7
White	107	16.0	25 – 29	144	21.5
Other	12	1.8	30 – 34	210	31.3
			35 – 39	136	20.3
SEX			40 – 44	58	8.7
Male	505	75.4	≥ 45	57	8.5
Female	165	24.6			
HOMELESSNESS (lifetime episodes)			PROBLEM SUBSTANCE(S) *		
Once	415	61.9	Multiple	352	52.5
Twice	100	14.9	Alcohol	319	47.6
Thrice	38	5.7	Crack	569	84.9
Four or more	117	17.5	Heroin	29	4.3
			Cannabis	67	10.0
EDUCATION (years completed)					
< 12	320	47.8			
12 – 16	346	51.6			
> 16	4	.6			
ALCOHOL TREATMENT HISTORY**			NON-ALCOHOL DRUG TREATMENT HISTORY**		
None	490	73.1	None	308	46.0
I – 2	109	16.3	I – 2	273	40.7
3 – 4	27	4.0	3 – 4	48	7.2
5 or more	44	6.6	5 or more	41	6.1

Self-reported and non-exclusive   **Prior times in treatment

DIAGRAM 1. – NOHSAP RESEARCH CLIENT FLOW (circa 9/15/92)

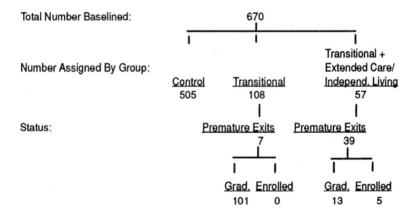

Total Number Baselined: 670

Number Assigned By Group:

Control   Transitional   Transitional + Extended Care/ Independ. Living
505   108   57

Status: Premature Exits   Premature Exits
               7   39

               Grad. Enrolled   Grad. Enrolled
               101   0   13   5

The first cohort of Extended Care clients has only recently graduated from the program and so there are insufficient follow-up data available to undertake even a preliminary analysis of program effectiveness. Three-month follow-ups document lower relapse rates among treatments than controls but we are not yet in a position to analyze other program outcomes. All program clients regardless of experimental status are assessed at three, six, and twelve months; a subset will also get an 18-month follow-up interview.

Initial three-month follow-up for the last baseline cohort will not occur until the end of July, 1992. To date, however, extensive tracking has yielded a three-month and six-month interview follow-up rate of 80%. Sample retention at the one-year mark has fallen, but only slightly to 75%. Through mid-July 1992, a total of 1324 follow-up interviews have been completed.

CONCLUSIONS AND IMPLICATIONS

Treatment for alcohol and drug disorders is difficult in the best of circumstances, and homelessness is assuredly not "the best of circumstances." Thus, we harbor no illusions about the ultimate results of the NOHSAP experiment. Many of our clients will leave our program as they entered it: broke, homeless, besotted, unkempt, with few or no prospects of a better life in the future. Given the relapse rates characteristic of alcohol and drug programs even for affluent people, however, it is clear that a program like NOHSAP does not have to be exceptionally effective to exceed any reasonable expectation. Here as in much of life, success is measured more by the distance travelled than by the destination reached, and if it turns out that only ten or twenty per cent of our clients succeed in getting their lives back together, that is still more than would have done so had they been left entirely to their own devices.

Jesus said, "So long as you did it to the least of mine, you did it unto me." There is no reasonable doubt that homeless alcoholics and drug addicts are "the least of mine," the very bottom of the urban poverty barrel. To have offered hope when before there was none is a worthwhile program accomplishment however modest the long term effects may ultimately prove to be.

REFERENCES

Aral, S. & Holmes, K. K. (1991). Sexually transmitted diseases in the AIDS era. *Scientific American, 264* (February), 62-69.

Brown, S. (1985). *Treating the alcoholic: a developmental model of recovery.* New York: John Wiley and Sons.

Children's Defense Fund. (1992). *Children in poverty, 1989.* Washington, DC: Children's Defense Fund.

Fisher, P. W., & Breakey, W. R. (1987). Profile of Baltimore homeless with alcohol problems. *Alcohol Health and Research World, 11* (3), 36-38.

Fisk, N. (1984). Epidemiology of alcohol abuse and alcoholism. *Alcohol Health and Research World, 9* (1), 4-7.

Homeless addicts get $3.1 million. (1990, October). New Orleans, *The Times-Picayune,* p. B-1.

Institute of Medicine. (1988). *Homelessness, health, and human needs.* Washington, DC: National Academy Press.

Koegel, P., & Burnham, M. A. (1987). Traditional and nontraditional homeless alcoholics. *Alcohol Health and Research World, 11* (3), 28-34.

Korenbaum, S., & Burney, G. (1987). Program planning for alcohol-free living centers. *Alcohol Health and Research World, 11* (3), 68-73.

Miller, M., Gorski, T., & Miller, D. (1982). *Learning to live again: a guide for recovery from alcoholism.* Independence, MO: Independence Press.

Ropers, R. H., & Boyer, R. (1987). Homelessness as a health risk. *Alcohol Health and Research World, 11* (3), 38-41.

Roth, D., & Bean, J. (1985). *Alcohol problems and homelessness: findings from the Ohio study.* Columbus, OH: Ohio Department of Mental Health, Office of Program Evaluation and Research.

U.S. Bureau of the Census. (1985). *Poverty areas in large cities.* [Subject reports PC80-2-8D.] Washington, DC: USGPO.

Wright, J. D. (1989a). *Address unknown: the homeless in America.* Hawthorne, NY: Aldine de Gruyter.

Wright, J. D. (1989b). *Correlates and consequences of alcohol abuse in the national "health care for the homeless" client population: final results.* Washington, DC: National Institute on Alcohol Abuse and Alcoholism.

Barriers to the Implementation of a Program for Inner-City, Homeless Substance Abusers on General Assistance: Newark

John Earl Franklin, MD
Jacob Jay Lindenthal, PhD, Dr PH
Meryl Sufian, PhD

SUMMARY. The article describes the implementation of a comprehensive rehabilitation program for homeless substance abusers within an inner-city setting. The program was a joint effort between a university research team and the general welfare department of the City of Newark, NJ. A description of the program is followed by a discussion of the political, economic, philosophical and bureaucratic barriers towards implementation of the project. Strengths and weaknesses of multiple agency efforts to rehabilitate homeless substance abusers are discussed. Complex systems issues that may be generalizable to other similar settings are highlighted. Conclusions and recommendations for implementation of future projects are presented.

John Earl Franklin is Assistant Professor of Clinical Psychiatry, Department of Psychiatry, UMDNJ-New Jersey Medical School. Jacob Jay Lindenthal is Professor, Department of Psychiatry, UMDNJ-New Jersey Medical School. Meryl Sufian is Project Director.
This work was supported by NIAAA grant 1U01AAA08783-1.

[Haworth co-indexing entry note]: "Barriers to the Implementation of a Program for Inner-City, Homeless Substance Abusers on General Assistance: Newark." Franklin, John Earl, Jacob Jay Lindenthal, and Meryl Sufian. Co-published simultaneously in the *Alcoholism Treatment Quarterly* (The Haworth Press, Inc.) Vol. 10, No. 3/4, 1993, pp. 65-76; and: *Treatment of the Chemically Dependent Homeless: Theory and Implementation in Fourteen American Projects* (ed: Kendon J. Conrad, Cheryl I. Hultman, and John S. Lyons) The Haworth Press, Inc., 1993, pp. 65-76. Multiple copies of this article/chapter may be purchased from The Haworth Document Delivery Center [1-800-3-HA-WORTH: 9:00 a.m. - 5:00 p.m. (EST)].

INTRODUCTION

The Newark, NIAAA Cooperative Agreement, Research Demonstration for Homeless Addicts was originated by the Division of Substance Abuse, Department of Psychiatry of the New Jersey Medical School, in close collaboration with the Department of Public Welfare of the City of Newark, Catholic Community Services, and a private housing developer. The target population is primarily African American and Latino men between the ages of 18 and 55 who receive general public assistance. To date, this has included 109 men with greater than 70% completion rate of the experimental interventions.

Newark is a Northeastern city of approximately 300,000 citizens. It is a city plagued with many of the problems that are facing other metropolitan areas including crime, drugs, unemployment, poor health care, substandard schools and a failed industrial base. There were approximately 5,000 individuals on the general assistance case load at the initiation of the granting period with 800 being on the homeless case load.

The magnitude and importance of the problems we have sought to address can be appreciated better when we consider that over one in every three of the homeless or 35 percent have alcohol disorders and an additional 15 to 20 percent have other drug disorders (National Resource Center on Homelessness and Mental Illness 1991) and that the prevalence of comorbidity for mental disorder in any one month period ranges from 37 percent among those with an alcohol disorder and 53 percent among those with other drug disorders (Regier et al., 1990). The odds ratio of those with mental illness having an addictive disorder was 2.7. Alcohol or other drug abusers had a seven fold greater probability of using the other addictive substance compared with the rest of the population.

Estimates indicate $11.54 in social costs are saved for every dollar spent on the treatment of drug abuse (National Association of Alcohol and Drug Abuse 1990) and that effective treatment of alcohol and drug abuse improves psychological adjustment, increases employment while decreasing crime and other forms of anti-social behavior (Tabbush 1986). One study in this vein found that among 10,000 individuals in treatment during a five year period, treatment returned to society almost the entire cost of the treatment during the same time with costs to society reduced by approximately 8 percent. The costs to victims of drug-related crime was reduced by about 30 percent, the criminal justice system about 24 percent and of theft, by 11 percent (National Institute on Drug Abuse 1989).

OBJECTIVES OF TREATMENT

The principal objective of the Newark project is to provide scientific data to assist program managers and providers to provide more comprehensive and efficient services for urban, homeless, substance abusing men; assisting them in recovery from substance abuse, attaining jobs and securing permanent housing. The objective is to create and understand the effectiveness of an innovative, comprehensive approach to providing drug/alcohol recovery emphasizing peer group cohesion, pre-vocational attitude and motivational training, specific skill training and placement activities in a well-ordered, sequential manner.

The design was a 2 by 2 factorial design with four experimental groups: (1) standard care; (2) enhanced vocational training and standard case management; (3) enhanced case management and standard vocational training; (4) enhanced case management and vocational training. The duration of the intervention was five to seven months.

To accomplish the primary objective of studying rehabilitation models with the target population, this project necessarily involved an attempt to institute a complicated psychosocial research design within a welfare population and system. Embedded in this attempt was the necessity of having the University community cooperate closely with the Newark, New Jersey, Department of Public Welfare.

THEORY OF TREATMENT

Four treatment models are employed in this project: case management, recovery, residential and vocational rehabilitation.

Case Management. Case management consists of two models: a standard or usual care approach initiated in the control group and an intense approach in the experimental group. The usual care approach consists of a large caseload, referrals with little follow-up, and client initiated contact with the case manager. The intensive case management approach utilizes an external, mixed use model focusing on coordination and linkage of service delivery with individual clients. The intense case management model consists of a small caseload, referrals made with frequent monitoring and client advocacy (Willenbring et al. 1991). The case manager has direct contact with clients as well as providers of services and is pro-active in initiating contact with clients.

Recovery Model. The recovery model that we are employing in this project is based on the following principles: (1) alcoholism and chemical dependency are chronic illnesses for which effective intervention/treatment exist; (2) self-help groups, and peer support and interaction are essential for a stable recovery from chemical dependency; and (3) the homeless with alcohol and drug problems can be taught to grow and change.

Residential Model. The residential model employed in this project is one that provides alcohol and drug-free housing to individuals who are homeless and recovering from chemical dependency. Our approach is based on the assumption that a living environment that is supportive to recovery values, customs, and rituals is a necessary substrate to provide a setting in which social skills can be developed for long term sobriety. The basic house philosophy is one of mutual self help, peer support, and confrontation of anti-social behavior as major tools within a model of recovery that sees a sociocultural environment as an important component to recovery.

This philosophy emphasizes the direct experiential knowledge gained from living in a drug-free community, taking responsibility for one's own personal recovery, learning from recovery role-models, and working with peers who are confronting similar recovery issues.

Vocational Model. The vocational model is based on a specialized training and employment program that utilizes the existing services at an established vocational center and is designed with specific modifications in training curricula and work adjustment for a recovering population. These modifications are designed to meet the needs of an inner-city ethnic minority recovering population consisting of individuals who are functioning on a variety of levels. Approaches to rehabilitation for this population can range from short-term job placement programs to long-term comprehensive rehabilitation efforts.

There are four phases in the vocational program: (1) orientation and evaluation, which includes the client's confronting their attitudes and past work performance; (2) entry level occupational skills training or advanced training modules tailored to the client's needs; (3) work adjustment including a group counseling component. Hands-on work experience training is provided, as is classroom instruction conducive to the clients' development of favorable attitudes toward work, establishment of regular work habits, attainment of experience in managing on-the-job problems, the development of self-confidence, and acquisition of the skills necessary to achieve a successful job search.

COLLABORATION AND CONTROL

The Welfare Director and the Principal Investigator of the grant simultaneously received copies of the RFA (Request for Applications) for the cooperative agreement sponsored by NIAAA and NIDA to study treatment interventions in homeless substance abusers. The Welfare Director had a general interest in research questions in this population, and also had successful experiences in obtaining service grants as exemplified by those deriving from the McKinney homeless grants. It was envisioned as a project that the university and the city of Newark would work on in close cooperation. A telephone call was made to the principal investigator expressing an interest that the university might respond to this grant proposal with the clear understanding that the proposal required academic personnel to conceive and write the proposal. It was also the understanding in the university that this particular application was to be a research demonstration project that was to be driven primarily by research design criteria and standards. This was a requirement of the NIAAA. There was a superficial understanding that the goals and the agenda for the project were the same. These blanket assumptions proved subsequently to form a major impediment for implementation and completion of the project. The question of whether this project was fundamentally a research grant that was recruiting welfare clients or one which was solely conceived to further a welfare reform agenda was an unresolved, poorly confronted issue that eventually resulted in an impasse.

It would be helpful perhaps at this juncture to describe the three key initiators of the grant since the personalities and agenda of these people would later interact to influence the implementation of the project. The director of the Newark Welfare Department was an African-American woman with a social work background, who had strong ties to Newark. On her own initiative she used the existing welfare regulations to set up a creative variety of shelters, evaluation units, a substance abuse unit within the welfare department and treatment, as well as training opportunities for clients. She had been given positive political marks for reducing the welfare case loads. In view of the fact she was a political appointee, she functioned often in an unforgiving political ambiance. Her style, keyed to both self-preservation, and her own notions of the structure, process and outcome of research into this afflicted population was to become problematic for the university team.

The Principal Investigator was an African-American psychiatrist with considerable clinical experience and expertise concerning substance abuse. This was his first research experience as a principal investigator which entailed considerable administrative skill. He did have a working knowledge of the population to be served, as well as experience in psychosocial research and with the assistance of other academicians in the department wrote the funded research grant.

The funding agency is the third leg of this tripod and at the pre-award site visit, several concerns were raised about who in fact was to lead this project. It became clear that the NIAAA, in view of having become involved in a cooperative agreement was to take a very active role in monitoring the Newark project. There were concerns expressed early about the complexity and feasibility of the design as well as whether the principal investigator was going to have the ability to drive the research agenda in light of the bureaucracy of the welfare system.

This grant was conceived and implemented in an unstable welfare reform climate. At the time that the grant was written several resources were then available or created by the welfare director to add to or support the clinical activities of the grant. Over the course of the grant several key welfare rules and regulations were amended, expected and unexpected administrative problems arose, and some resources evaporated.

Despite the problems that will be highlighted in the following sections, the project was successful in recruitment of subjects, developing the basic service components, retaining clients and completing the research documentation. Several aspects of the grant worked extremely well. These barriers and successful aspects of the grant will be highlighted in the following sections.

FACILITIES

The funding for the service components of the grant initially derived from the city of Newark and NIAAA funding. These included housing, monies for 28 day rehabilitation, vocational training, case management and clinical supervision of the housing facility. The city was responsible under regulations to provide temporary shelter to people who came to their agency, lived in Newark and had no place to stay. They were placed typically in a 30 day emergency shelter and then transferred subsequently to a transitional facility for six months. Funding for the housing was obtained from the state and administered by the city of Newark.

The project looked at several potential sites and decided to employ an existing transitional shelter for the housing component of the grant. The constraints placed on the project team by the city regarding the housing site were later to cause difficulty for the design implementation. To minimize contamination among the four experimental groups the housing component needed to create four largely independent living areas. The project was constrained to the use of only one structure which consisted of a building with four floors and mirrored stairwells. The structure has a previous reputation for being a drug and alcohol infested building. It is surrounded physically by barbed wire and is located on a busy drug traffic block.

The plan was to effect minimal structural changes in order to create four independent living areas for 15 men each and provide needed security to keep undesirable influences from the building. There were strongly harbored differences with respect for the need to control the building with security personnel. The issues of control were to develop into a major source of differences in philosophy between the clinical and research staff at the university and the city welfare department. The bureaucracy of the welfare department appeared to be concerned primarily with control of the clientele and the issues of process which impinged on the agreed upon scientific program. Differences on the issue of control of the clients and of process issues proved to be an impediment to the resolution of some of the problems. It became evident very early that there was a push and pull between the needs of the research design, the financial interests of the developers and the City's need to avoid the NIMBY (not in my backyard) syndrome.

The developer expressed concrete fears that by investing too heavily in this facility in order to fit the specifications of the project, he might expose this facility to too much public scrutiny. The result was a difficult, uneasy, retarded negotiation process in extracting the required structural changes despite assurances that the grant was able to pay for renovations.

Several rehabilitation facilities were contacted and expressed interest in treating the clients with the understanding that it was to be under the auspices of the state and the NIAAA research demonstration grant. Representatives of the rehabilitation facilities expressed indirectly some reservations about servicing a homeless population but also welcomed the possible referral base. The eight facilities chosen were all state rehabilitation facilities and were all well respected facilities employing standard inpatient approaches to treatment which included for the most part, domiciled, insurance or Medicaid clients. Initial fears that the homeless subgroups of 5-10 clients would not integrate well into the treatment milieu proved to be unfounded. The uniform response from the facilities was that these clients were well motivated, cooperative and an asset to the groups with only a few exceptions.

The Boland vocational facility is geographically located near the university, the welfare office and the transition house. The welfare director had discussed previously with the director of the vocational facility the possibility of sending some of her clients to that facility for training. The vocational facility was primarily an agency that serviced physically, mentally challenged and geriatric clients. The challenge for the project was being able to adapt their structure to the needs of our population. The facility had no specific experience with the rehabilitation of substance abusers or homeless clients.

A number of efforts were made by NIAAA and its consultants (ROW Sciences) to expose the agency to prior work done in the field and provided contacts and models of treatment upon which the agency might draw. There remained throughout the grant a tendency towards inflexibility and paucity of creativity on the part of the vocational staff in adapting their rehabilitation philosophy to the needs of the clients. In the end however, vocational modules were devised that fit the varied needs of the clientele. Vocational tracks included in-house training and outside schools or training programs that were suitable to individual clients and fit the research design. It should be noted that several scheduling conflicts arose between the bureaucratic needs of retaining welfare eligibility and the training schedule. These scheduling problems impacted negatively on the progress of the project. In addition, extensive delays were incurred in the vocational component while the welfare department sought to determine from the state whether clients could be paid for their work. Outside work contracts ultimately had to be changed to in-house training projects.

The last major funding needed for the service component was for the case management which experienced the most convolution in both funding and conceptualization. The experience that derived from the previous clinical work the university and city had conducted with this population had highlighted the lacunae into which clients fall without adequate case management. The research question became the following: What is adequate or optimal case management for welfare clients who are homeless and abusing drugs.

The design in both its original and resolved forms intended to test the differences between enhanced and more standard welfare case management. The city of Newark at the time of the implementation of the grant was in the midst of a hiring freeze. No employee could be hired by the city to work on this project even if the funds for a position could be derived from the grant budget. This created a fundamental dilemma. The project needed a case worker who would have access to the DPW system to be able to handle the myriad service vouchers and certification requirements. To be able to have access to the welfare system the case worker was required to be a civil service employee. The inability to subcontract with the city for services and to formalize the expectations of cooperation from this agency proved to be a problem in the administration of the project.

It became evident that despite efforts on the part of the university as well as of the national evaluation team of the NIAAA to explain the problems inherent in the psychosocial research process and to assure a fair test of the hypotheses generated, representatives of the city differed on how to implement some key elements of the research design. We have rediscovered the importance of keeping senior officials at both the city and state levels of government well informed on the progress of the project.

COORDINATING COMMITTEE

There was a several month start up period to the grant. As research training was conducted on the national level, hiring was taking place and operationalization was discussed. These deliberations were always done in committee involving the P.I., co-P.I.'s and service providers. An unfortunate blurring of roles developed between researchers and providers. Several members of the study doubled as both clinical directors and research investigators. The committee approach to decisions was for the most part an inefficient, tedious, and sometimes acrimonious process primarily because of differences in the fundamental approach or model of handling clients as envisioned by the welfare system, the clinical personnel and the constraints of the research design. The welfare system is set up to process a large number of clients through a bureaucratic system and measures success by its ability to function smoothly. The clinical approach to these patients required decisions based on what was considered in the best interests of the individual and group milieu necessary to foster growth and development. The research design demanded a clear set of interventions that could be tested in a quasi-experimental fashion. After considerable work, it was generally acknowledged that there would need to be compromises to accomplish this "real world" psychosocial research.

STAFFING

The differences in philosophy were evident when the project director was hired. Several potential project directors were presented to the service providers for review and commentary. The backgrounds of the PhD level applicants ranged from strengths in biostatistics and research design, field work on similar psychosocial projects to one candidate whose chief strength was as a hospital administrator. The research team had a strong preference for the candidates with a prior background in population psychosocial research. The service providers identified and felt most trustful of the administrator who planned to provide a strong administrative hand. Some disagreement ensued in which the service providers were reluctant to cooperate with the university team unless the administrator was hired.

The strengths that this person, whom they hired, possessed helped secure the confidence of the welfare director and the director of the vocational facility but diminished when the welfare director did not feel that the project was collaborating with service providers fully enough. In addition, some frustration was expressed by the service providers with the NIAAA project staff because they were sometimes seen as intrusive and not sensitive to service providers needs. The initial project director was eventually replaced partly due to the service providers insistence. Some momentum was lost as it took time to hire another project director.

It was also recognized that the project housing component would need clinical supervision and staffing. These monies were designated to be included in the service component portion of the grant. Several full time and half time personnel were hired to fill these clinical slots. A major disagreement developed between the university management and the city regarding qualifications and suitability of the house manager. The welfare department was interested in hiring a person who would be very responsive to welfare bureaucratic needs. The house manager was seen as someone who would maintain order with the clients rather than be a facilitator of a self-help process. The university was more concerned with creating a recovery atmosphere in the house. An African-American recovering man with a background in managing a half way house for addicts, and a potential role model, was favored by the university staff. A man who had extensive experience in the prison system was preferred by the welfare director. The hiring of this key position in addition to the project director were symbols of crucial differences in philosophy and management style between the welfare system and the clinical staff.

Members of the NIAAA staff harbored concerns about the potential problems of the working arrangement between the university and the city from the inception of the project. It was felt generally that it was going to be difficult to extract the flexibility and cooperation needed from the city to maintain a tight research design. The NIAAA staff also had reservations about the eventual resolution of some of the more thorny differences in philosophy between the university and the city systems. It was felt that the P.I. needed to be strong to work with the service providers and provide leadership in the way of having a clear say regarding major decisions.

REVIEW AND REVISION

Reviews provided at the first year site visit by the NIAAA emphasized many of the above difficulties in the implementation of the project. Continued funding was tied to a very detailed action plan that was implemented successfully over a three month period. It entailed consultation with experts in the field, a significant design change to simplify the design, hiring of a new project director who would meet with the approval of NIAAA, the creation of a clearer organizational chart and better delineation of responsibilities. A follow-up site visit was arranged in which the reorganization plan was approved and agreed to by all parties. There was an unfortunate two month delay in fully implementing the new design changes because of budget complications. At the time of the March 1992 NIAAA site visit, the NIAAA staff congratulated the research staff on their significant progress in making impressive changes in the organization of the project, clarifying and strengthening the interventions, and the leadership role that the P.I. and project director were playing on the project. At the concluding meeting, the site team complimented project staff on their implementation of the recommendations made during the November 7-8, 1991 follow-up site visit which resulted in distinct qualitative improvements and an increased feeling of team spirit and client empowerment.

Prior to the March 1992 site visit however, the welfare director expressed continued frustration at the lack of progress in resolving some of the philosophical differences in management styles between the research staff and the city. It became apparent that significant welfare reform changes at the state level were eventually going to challenge the continuation of the project in its mature design. However, it was unclear at the time as to its immediate impact on the study. In addition, the welfare director subsequently left her position at the city in late May 1992 to spearhead a state welfare reform effort. The project ended prematurely after the second year of funding as it became clear that the feasibility was poor of completing the third year's goals of the project.

IMPLICATIONS FOR PRACTICE, RESEARCH, AND POLICY

Despite the myriad problems in the Newark project, the university staff and political leaders at the city, state, and federal levels remain enthusiastic about the mission of helping homeless with substance abuse problems. This group feels Newark can harvest the experience of the first two years of this project and capitalize on it. Discussions have begun on new initiatives to service and research this population. In the course of discussing the first two year's experience with this project, several recommendations will inform future grant efforts. Many of the recommendations are not new, but reconfirmed by the Newark project.

First, structured discussions between city and researchers should be undertaken prior to grant submission to have parties understand the culture in which each functions and from which each derives. These discussions have to lead to written agreements of sufficient detail to create esprit de corp between institutions in which each feels validated and protected as to its primary mission. Second, a community advisory board is essential to the process of this kind of grant to provide advice, support and cross community representation, and to minimize negative personality conflicts. Third, there must be real support of these kinds of projects from the mayor's office, city council and the health and human services director of the state. Fourth, federal funding agencies should not become involved in the collaborative process to the point of splitting local agencies that have to work with one another. Fifth, researchers have to be able to subcontract city and state agencies to protect the integrity of the research design.

The problems experienced in implementing this complex project are far outweighed by the success in recruiting subjects, the development of quality services, retention and graduation of better than expected numbers of people and satisfaction of seeing people get sober and renew a sense of hope for their lives. The accomplishments achieved by the project are due to the shared efforts of the services providers, NIAAA, the university staff and the clients.

REFERENCES

National Association of Alcohol and Drug Abuse Directors (1990, March). *Treatment Works.*

National Institute on Drug Abuse (1989, October). *Treatment Outcome Prospective Study.*

National Resource Center on Homelessness and Mental Illness. Access (1991, January) (3) 1.

Regier, D., Farmer, M.E. and Rae, Donald S. et al. (1990, November). Comorbidity of mental disorders with alcohol and other drug abuse: Results from the epidemiologic catchment area (ECA) study. *Journal of the American Medical Association* (264) 19:2511-2518.

Tabbush, V. (1986, March). *The Effectiveness and Efficiency of Publicly Funded Drug Abuse Treatment and Prevention Programs in California: A Benefit-Cost Analysis.* University of California, Los Angeles.

Willenbring, M., Ridgely, M., Stinchfield, R., and Rose, M. (1991, February). *Application of Case Management in Alcohol and Drug Dependence: Matching Techniques and Populations.* U.S. Department of Health and Human Services: Homeless Demonstration and Evaluation Branch.

Partnerships in Recovery: Shelter-Based Services for Homeless Cocaine Abusers: New Haven

Philip J. Leaf, PhD
Kenneth S. Thompson, MD
Julie A. Lam, PhD
James F. Jekel, MD, MPH
Esther T. Armand
Arthur E. Evans, PhD
John S. Martinez

Carmen Rodriguez
Wesley C. Westman, PhD
Paul Johnston, PhD
Michael Rowe, MPA
Stephanie Hartwell, MA
Howard Blue
Toni Harp

SUMMARY. The Grant Street Partnership (GSP) is a new, community-developed, shelter-based program of clinical and case-management services for homeless, cocaine-abusing men in New Haven,

---

Philip J. Leaf is affiliated with the Johns Hopkins School of Hygiene and Public Health; Kenneth S. Thompson is affiliated with Western Psychiatric Institute & Clinic; Julie A. Lam and James F. Jekel are both affiliated with Yale University School of Medicine, Department of Epidemiology & Public Health; Esther T. Armand and Arthur E. Evans are both affiliated with South Central Rehabilitation Center; John S. Martinez and Wesley C. Westman are both affiliated with Hill Health Center, Grant Street Partnership; Carmen Rodriguez is affiliated with the City of New Haven; Paul Johnston, Michael Rowe, and Stephanie Hartwell are all affiliated with Yale University, Department of Sociology.

Address correspondence to: Philip J. Leaf, Professor, Department of Mental Hygiene, Johns Hopkins School of Hygiene and Public Health, 624 North Broadway, Baltimore, MD 21205.

[Haworth co-indexing entry note]: "Partnerships in Recovery: Shelter-Based Services for Homeless Cocaine Abusers: New Haven." Leaf, Philip J. et al. Co-published simultaneously in the *Alcoholism Treatment Quarterly* (The Haworth Press, Inc.) Vol. 10, No. 3/4, 1993, pp. 77-90; and: *Treatment of the Chemically Dependent Homeless: Theory and Implementation in Fourteen American Projects* (ed: Kendon J. Conrad, Cheryl I. Hultman, and John S. Lyons) The Haworth Press, Inc., 1993, pp. 77-90. Multiple copies of this article/chapter may be purchased from The Haworth Document Delivery Center [1-800-3-HAWORTH: 9:00 a.m. - 5:00 p.m. (EST)].

Connecticut. The first component of the GSP is a 90-day residential program in which residents progress from one level of accomplishment and responsibility to the next, culminating in an assisted search for suitable housing and for employment or job training. Upon completion of the residential component, the clients continue in case management and clinical services for approximately six months on an ambulatory basis. The GSP has a second agenda of being an agent for improvement of housing, employment, and job-training services in New Haven. Because a wide spectrum of city institutions were involved in the development of the GSP, the partnership thus developed has continued and is being redirected toward institutional change of the type needed by the GSP clients.

INTRODUCTION

As with the other programs described in this volume, the Grant Street Partnership (GSP) is part of a large multi-site collaborative study administered by the National Institute of Alcohol Abuse and Alcoholism. The goal of the GSP is to provide a short-term shelter and day treatment program for homeless cocaine abusers in the City of New Haven. Thus, this program represents one of the first attempts to address specifically the problem of cocaine use among the homeless, a problem that co-occurs frequently with alcohol abuse. The program differs from the others described in this volume in at least three important ways.

First, the GSP was developed to meet the needs of homeless men who are primarily cocaine abusers, although most also use and often abuse other illegal drugs and alcohol. Most of the other programs described in this volume began with a focus on the alcohol problems of the homeless. Therefore, the target population of the Grant Street Partnership differs in a number of ways from the target population of the other programs described in this volume. For example, GSP clients tend to be younger and probably are more likely to have criminal histories.

A second difference is a matter of scale. New Haven, with a 1990 population of 130,474, is the smallest city included in the collaborative study and the only city that is not one of the nation's 40 largest. In addition to developing the GSP, persons affiliated with the program actively participate in city-wide efforts to deal with problems of violence, drug abuse, vocational training, and housing, giving the program a position of community leadership. Developers of the GSP recognized that community action was required if the GSP was to be successful. Also, the GSP is part of an organizational ecosystem, in which activities addressing one issue not only create change but also create pressure for other components of the system to change.

From the start, the program was constituted as a coalition with participation from the Office of the Mayor and the Board of Aldermen; local nongovernmental agencies such as the Hill Health Center; the South Central Rehabilitation Center; the Addiction Prevention and Treatment (APT) Foundation; Yale University; and the Connecticut Mental Health Center. This coalition allowed the GSP to overcome a series of obstacles to its inception that included: (1) developing a structure for accessing startup funds; (2) difficulties in procuring a site for the shelter; (3) a greatly delayed opening of the only local detoxification center; and (4) a budgetary crisis within the City of New Haven and the State of Connecticut. From the start, the program was seen as a flagship for change.

The third way this project differs from most of the other NIAAA projects is that GSP was a brand new agency. Since GSP did not exist prior to the receipt of the federal funds, preparations for opening the program were made very rapidly. Four months prior to the opening of the shelter, the building housing GSP had been a warehouse and the first staff not yet hired. In contrast to many of the programs reviewed in this issue, the GSP was a totally new program, in new "space," managed by an agency (the Hill Health Center) that had never before provided residential services. The entire program needed to be developed from scratch, and a new staff hired. The program has experienced the full range of problems that plague the development of new organizations. The birth of a new organization is never easy. Still, at an early developmental phase, GSP continues to grow and change. The remainder of this paper will describe the project, tracing its development and elaborating on its current status.

BACKGROUND

New Haven, like most cities in the U.S., experienced a rise in homelessness during the 1980s as jobs left Connecticut and single occupancy dwellings were converted into apartments to generate greater income. Unlike many cities, the New Haven Board of Aldermen did not succumb to the "not in my backyard" opposition of local residents. Rather, the Board developed a comprehensive city-wide program to address the emerging problems of the homeless in the City. This program included: the development of increased permanent low income housing and single room occupancy (SRO) units in scattered sites; increased support for emergency housing; the appointment of a city-wide homeless coordinator; and regional cooperation to address the problems of homelessness in south central Connecticut.

At the same time that the number of homeless was increasing, New

Haven experienced an increase in the use of crack cocaine. The substance abuse treatment system, already overwhelmed, was unable to respond to the increased demand for services. The epidemic threatened the viability of the existing system of city-financed shelters.

The idea for the GSP first surfaced at a meeting of the Aldermanic Committee on the Homeless, which was chaired by the Director of the Health Care for the Homeless Program operated by the Hill Health Center. A coalition consisting of staff from the agencies noted previously met to consider a variety of options for furthering the Homeless Housing Plan that had been developed by the City's Board of Aldermen in July 1989. A proposal had already been submitted to the State for capital funds to convert the first floor of a factory on Grant Street for use as a shelter and day program, but the City's projected budget deficit of $30 million meant that no resources existed for operating the new facility if it were constructed. The proposal to the NIAAA, therefore, emerged as a vehicle to provide the City with staffing for a facility that they were willing to rehabilitate, to provide the Hill Health Center with resources to expand their program of health care for the homeless to include comprehensive shelter-based and aftercare services for homeless men with substance abuse problems. The proposal also provided an opportunity for faculty at Yale University to test a model of shelter-based services for the homeless that evolved out of their experiences with services for homeless persons in other communities.

From the start, the program involved negotiation and political tradeoffs. For example, City officials made it clear that they needed to provide beds for more than the 25 individuals to be included in the research project proposed by the Yale researchers. In the end, it was agreed that the GSP would contain 44 beds and that 19 of these beds would be for homeless men who were not substance abusers. There was also debate concerning the duration of the allowable shelter residence. This was set at 90 days. The service providers wished for a longer period of residence, but the City desired the shortest possible duration because the State would provide funding only for short-term shelters and because the City officially had no wish to get into the business of providing long-term residences to the homeless at a time of fiscal crisis. Thus, the 90 day residence established for the study was a compromise, and its effectiveness needs careful evaluation.

The role of the researchers in the project also has been the subject of ongoing negotiation and compromise. Possibly because New Haven is one of the most thoroughly researched cities in the nation, community leaders and service providers feel that they are more frequently the research subjects of, rather than collaborators with, researchers at Yale University. Because the senior researchers at Yale were white and the majority of community collaborators and potential clients were African-American or Hispanic, potential exploitation was the subject of more than one discussion. From the project's inception, the Executive Committee constantly struggled with the need to balance the concerns of community providers for relevance, the interests of the researchers in "rigor," and the concerns of governmental representatives regarding cost. The compromises made by all and the continued existence of the program attests to the level of trust that evolved from these discussions.

The development of the GSP, however, was not all compromise. All those participating in the Grant Street Partnership made contributions to developing and sustaining the program through a series of crises that would have devastated a program with less solidarity and less community support. City officials facilitated the site approval by neighborhood residents and identified local residents to serve on a neighborhood advisory board to ensure that concerns of local residents would be dealt with expeditiously. Interestingly, the first concerns raised by the neighborhood oversight committee were about the privacy of the residents at the GSP and the quality of their food and health care. When sale of the factory building put the entire project in jeopardy, local officials moved the negotiations ahead.

Another example of teamwork occurred when the opening of the detoxification program, a key component of the program and the site of randomization for the study, was substantially delayed. Rather than jeopardizing the success of the project, staff at the South Central Rehabilitation Corporation (SCRC) created a "bridge" program (described below) by negotiating expedited entry into detoxification facilities located in other distant communities and accepting responsibility for transportation to and from the detoxification facility.

Similarly, without the confidence that the homeless men and shelter operators had in the Hill Health Center's Health Care for the Homeless Team, the tight schedule for integrating the new GSP into the existing shelter network would have been impossible. Finally, the Yale University School of Medicine expedited funding of subcontracts so that the Hill Health Center's cash flow would not be burdened by the new initiative. The GSP continues to be guided by an interagency executive committee which includes the staff from the program, the research team, local agencies, and the Mayor's office.

ASSESSING THE NEED

Once funding was obtained for the project, the executive committee of the GSP needed additional information about the potential clients for the new program. The target population–homeless cocaine abusers–was originally selected after conversations with providers of services to the homeless in New Haven. In order to obtain a better description of the target population, and to obtain the views of potential participants concerning service needs, a survey was conducted of the five emergency shelters in New Haven during a four-week interval in November and December 1990 (Spinner and Leaf, 1992). At the time of the survey, these shelters provided little beyond a bed and a meal. This survey of 181 homeless persons found that during the 30 days before the interview 53% of the respondents had used alcohol to intoxication, 41% had used cocaine, and 27% had used marijuana.

Two-thirds of the homeless persons identified substance use as a reason for their homelessness, and approximately one-third of the shelter respondents reported drug-related criminal activity. This is probably an underestimate, but it does suggest that an important community benefit to substance treatment programs for the homeless might be a reduction in thefts and drug-related violence.

Only 44% of the respondents reported any previous treatment for a drug or alcohol problem. Their substance abuse contributed both to the potential clients' loss of housing and their inability to sustain housing. Thus, the conclusions of previous informal needs assessments were supported by the survey, and considerable data were obtained for planning the program and scheduling activities for the new shelter. The survey did not, however, determine the number of homeless substance abusers who would be willing to commit to a 3-month period of restricted residence, nor the procedures for identifying homeless substance abusers who were ready to enter the program.

In addition to the survey, an extensive effort was made to conduct qualitative research examining how potential clients might view the project and what features they would like to see in a drug treatment program. Unstructured interviews as well as focus groups were conducted with substance abusers residing in city shelters. Such topics as the content and structure of the program, the name of the program, and cultural issues were discussed extensively, and many of the men's ideas were incorporated into the Grant Street Partnership.

THE GRANT STREET PARTNERSHIP

The GSP was created to achieve two different but related goals. The first was to establish a shelter-based program of services for New Haven's cocaine-abusing homeless men. The program was unable to provide services to women because of the physical layout of the building and the inability to provide services to the children who live with these women. The second goal was to expand existing services that were needed by homeless individuals or to collaborate in developing new services, such as employment and transitional housing that were not currently available or easily accessible to homeless individuals in New Haven.

The actual substance abuse treatment program at the GSP consists of two major components. The first is a 90-day residential program operated in a 24-hour shelter. It is located in a former munitions factory, the first floor of which was rehabilitated with funds from the State of Connecticut and purchased by the City of New Haven. The renovations, while aesthetically pleasing, were of relatively low cost, due to the creativity of the architects and contractors.

RECRUITMENT OF CLIENTS

In the original plan, most of the GSP clients were to be referred from the detoxification facilities operated by a new program, South Central Rehabilitation Center (SCRC), whose director was involved in the planning of the GSP from the beginning. Originally scheduled to open in the Spring of 1991, this facility has not yet opened its detoxification program, which greatly complicated the problems of client recruitment for the project. This crisis, however, also forced the GSP to confront the issue of recruitment/outreach and to develop a program to inform the potential clients and service providers about the GSP.

SCRC hired a full-time outreach worker to inform the staff at the other shelters of the new program and to transport clients to and from detoxification units elsewhere. So far, most clients of the GSP have been referred from existing homeless shelters in New Haven. Additional outreach efforts have been made at the soup kitchens, hospitals, and with the criminal justice system. Thus, the recruitment process became a key component of treatment initiation.

Potential clients for the evaluation study are screened for eligibility for the study while at the detoxification facility. The screening criteria are that the men must be 18 years of age or older, from the New Haven metropolitan area, currently homeless or marginally housed and at risk of becoming homeless, and have a history of or current problem with cocaine use. Exclusionary criteria include the existence of a physical illness requiring more care than can be provided at the shelter, active psychoses, and extremely disruptive or violent behavior while in detox. After the men meet the screening criteria they are informed about the study and asked to consent to randomization into either the GSP or standard community services. Originally, all potential clients were first sent to a detoxification facility for 3-5 days, where they were interviewed and then randomized to either the GSP or "usual services" by staff employed by the research component of this project. Following detoxification, the study participants were then transported to either the GSP or one of the other shelters in New Haven. Although this process enabled the GSP to obtain clients, it was somewhat erratic and complex in implementation. Often men would leave the detoxification facility prior to the research interview.

Increasingly, clients have come directly from shelters without going to a detoxification facility, providing they pass the physical examination and have drug-free urine. These men are required to be on "stay-in" status at the shelter for 3 to 5 days prior to the interview and randomization to help ensure that they are free of drugs. This has increased the flow of men into the GSP.

THE RESIDENTIAL PROGRAM

The GSP itself is a monitored, drug-free, 24-hour shelter where clients are introduced into a modified therapeutic community with a levels program involving increasingly greater responsibilities and privileges. The shelter-based component of the program lasts for approximately 90 days. Upon arriving at the shelter, clients are assigned a case manager. After an assessment and evaluation, clients and case managers develop an individualized substance abuse treatment contract and service plan aimed at achieving and maintaining abstinence and accessing the services necessary to facilitate integration into the community. While case management has been increasingly used with other populations, it is a new concept in substance abuse treatment (Sullivan et al., 1992; Timney and Graham, 1989). The program at the shelter consists of both individual and group activities. The men are involved in a coordinated program of activities aimed at improving daily living skills, developing self expression skills, creating a drug-free social network, and fostering a sense of individual and group empowerment and self-determination. Twelve step programming has been thoroughly incorporated into this program as well. In addition, health problems are identified during an intake examination conducted by staff from the Hill Health Center. Any medical care necessary is provided by the HHC.

The shelter-based component of the program involves three levels: orientation, resource acquisition, and re-entry. In level one, the resident becomes acquainted with the program and its requirements, undergoes a psychosocial evaluation, is assigned a "Big Brother" who is another resident, begins meetings with his case manager and other program staff to develop a service plan, and begins daily group counseling and psychosocial groups. The individual participates in AA/NA meetings within the shelter. In addition, a program of individual counseling is established.

In level two the individual can become a "Big Brother" to incoming residents, can receive weekend passes, and has telephone privileges. Participation continues in group and individual programs and the resident is involved in a variety of activities such as the maintenance of the shelter facility and outside AA/NA meetings. He begins to focus on implementing the service plan, especially issues related to employment and housing. In level three, the resident develops plans for maintaining in his community his educational, employment, and other commitments, opens a savings account, and develops an aftercare plan with his case manager. Residents at all levels meet weekly together in a "town meeting" to discuss programmatic issues. Program graduates sometimes speak at the town meetings and frequently return for "graduations."

The program also has attempted to be sensitive to ethnic and racial factors that might influence the effectiveness of the program and the attractiveness of the program to clients. The program has a multi-racial executive committee and staff, with several of the staff being bilingual. The psychiatric consultant for the program is an African-American. Discussions of race and ethnicity occur frequently in the context of the program. There is an ongoing effort to establish links with the formal and informal leaders of the neighborhoods to which most of the men return. The GSP also attempts to reconnect the men with their families, parents, siblings, wives, and children.

THE AFTERCARE PROGRAM

Following discharge from the shelter, a six-month program of supervised case-management and group activities at the GSP is to be made available to each client. This component of the program has proven to be more difficult to establish. Originally, staff were to have responsibility for case management of both residents and graduates of the shelter program, but staff have had difficulty diverting their attention from clients in the shelter, and, therefore, the six-month case management component has consisted primarily of telephone contacts and brief meetings between staff and graduates. This does not provide sufficient treatment and support for the graduates, especially given the high levels of drug use and violence in the neighborhoods where most of the available housing exists. The inadequate number of community treatment, training, and employment opportunities presents a serious challenge both to the recovering addict and to the staff. Recently, however, the program has achieved some success with men moving into "clean" group apartments.

THE EVALUATION STUDY

The GSP is being evaluated by a randomized design in which applicants who meet the admission criteria, and who agree to be a part of the research, are randomized either to the GSP or to "customary community care," which consists of homeless shelters with some case management, AA and NA programs in the community, outpatient substance abuse treatment programs affiliated with Yale University, and several other residential detoxification and treatment programs including the Salvation Army Adult Rehabilitation program. Currently there are only two homeless shelters in New Haven serving the men in our study. Men who are not randomized into GSP are connected with a case manager at one of the shelters. The existing programs overlap with the GSP only in the sense that they provide shelter and in some cases, very limited case management with large caseloads. The shelter case managers begin to work on alternative treatment possibilities for the men even before the research interview in anticipation that they might not be randomized into GSP.

To date, the program has had too few clients and controls complete the 9-month program to assess the long-term impact on individuals. Impressionistic indicators of success are that there have been no serious incidents in the shelter involving any man actively participating in the program, and a strong sense of "family" exists in the facility. In addition, the retention rate of clients has been improving.

As indicated earlier, the shelter-based activities of the GSP constitute one of a two-pronged strategy. In addition to the GSP, staff and others associated with the program have been involved in increasing the awareness of the local community of the need for additional housing and treatment services for homeless men. They have probably had their major impact in strengthening the Common Ground program, a pre-vocational training program funded by the Private Industry Council, into which several GSP graduates have been accepted. The purpose of this program is to bring the client's level of education and skills to a point where they can make good use of the existing job training programs. The GSP also has stimulated activities aimed at providing relief for individuals on general assistance in the city, which includes most of the participants in the GSP.

Although progress in each of these areas has been slow, there has been a definite shift in the City's agenda. Efforts to reduce the use of substances, to reduce the level of shootings and other violence, to increase housing, and to provide additional job training for residents of the inner city are now being addressed. Many of these discussions have been precipitated by the efforts of the Grant Street Partnership and the groundwork that preceded it. Whether these efforts will persist and achieve success remains to be seen.

Study Subjects

While the impact of the project on clinical outcomes of patients is unknown, a clearer sense of the GSP clients is emerging. Through April of 1992, 110 men had participated in the NIAAA Cooperative Agreement which included the Grant Street Partnership. Of these men, 82 were in the experimental group and 28 were in the control group. The original research plan called for the randomization of equal numbers of homeless cocaine abusers to the GSP and the existing community programs. Randomization was suspended for two months during the fall, however, because the initial recruitment into the GSP was not rapid enough to produce a critical number of clients required for the efficient operation of the program. The lack of residents created a feeling of emptiness within the shelter that affected both the residents and the staff. Late in the fall, randomization was reinstated, but the ratio of persons assigned to the Grant Street Shelter was modified from time to time to keep the number of residents high enough to allow for the conduct of the programming. Due to the increasing reputation of GSP in the community and to increased recruitment efforts, numbers are not currently a problem at GSP and the ratio may be changed so as to increase the proportion of control subjects.

Changes in the randomization procedures did not affect the equivalence of the two groups, however. Tests conducted on baseline data from the two groups revealed no statistically significant nor programmatically important differences on any of the key demographic or life history variables. Therefore, the characteristics reported below are for both groups combined.

PRELIMINARY FINDINGS

The data provide interesting insights into the problems and life experiences of homeless cocaine abusing men. The average age was 31 years. The majority of subjects were African Americans, most had not completed high school, had never been married, and had lived alone when they were not in a homeless shelter. Most had not been born in the New Haven area but had lived in New Haven more than half their lives.

The men participating in this study were not the chronically, long-term homeless. During the 60 days prior to being randomized, the average number of nights spent in an emergency shelter was 23, and none had spent time in a public place, bus, abandoned building, car, or outdoor place. The average number of times homeless was 2.6 and the average age when they first became homeless was 27, or approximately four years prior to randomization. The men typically used the emergency shelters as places to seek safety or respite from difficult situations, which were usually due either to their drug use, their home life, or both. Only 11 percent of the men had had no stable living arrangement during the previous year.

Over two-thirds of the men had usually been employed during the previous year, but almost three-quarters of the men had not worked for pay during the 30 days prior to entering the program. The average total income from all sources (including illegal) during the 30 days prior to detoxification was just under $1,000 ($958.28).

Regarding substance abuse, 91% said that they had used cocaine or crack in the 30 days prior to detoxification (and all had histories of cocaine abuse); the average number of days of use during these 30 days was 17, and the average number of years of regular cocaine use was seven. The men were most likely to smoke cocaine (54%), followed by intravenous use (29%), snorting or sniffing (15%), and injecting non-intravenously (3%). The men were generally multi-substance users with 76% also using alcohol, 33% using heroin or P-Dope (a synthetic drug similar to heroin and often used interchangeably), 27% using marijuana, and 24% injecting speedballs (heroin and cocaine combined) in the 30 days prior to detoxification.

The average number of previous treatments for alcohol abuse was 1.8 and the average number for drug abuse was 2.3. The men were more likely to have reported problems with drugs in the past 30 days (18.4 days on average) than with alcohol (10.3 days on average).

Just over one-quarter of the men had a chronic medical problem: 13% with high blood pressure and 10% with sexually transmitted diseases, including HIV. Mental health problems plague a significant minority of the men, with 16% having been hospitalized overnight for a psychological problem and 18.2% having received outpatient psychological treatment. Nineteen percent of the men had attempted suicide at some point in their lives. Evidence gathered in structured psychiatric interviews (SCID) done on each man at the GSP demonstrated a high rate of clinical and subclinical depression, in the context of long histories of social and family disruption, especially related to poverty and parental substance abuse. Psychoses were relatively uncommon, probably due to the process of recruitment. Most of the depressed men appear to improve spontaneously when in the shelter.

Four out of five study participants had been arrested and charged with a crime at least once as an adult (80.2%). The average number of times arrested and charged with a crime was 6.2, with an average of 4.6 of these arrests resulting in convictions. The largest number of men had drug-related arrests (41.4%), followed by burglary, larceny, or breaking and entering (40.5%). In addition, over half (51.8%) had been arrested for disorderly conduct, vagrancy, or public drunkenness. Nearly three-quarters of the men had spent two weeks or more incarcerated in a jail, prison, or detention center. The average length of incarceration was just over two years (24.9 months). Nearly one-quarter of the men were on parole or probation at the time of the baseline interview.

CONCLUSION

While it is too early to determine the effectiveness of the GSP on improving the outcomes of the men, it is possible to say that the program has already had a significant impact on the way that the City of New Haven approaches the problem of homelessness. It has helped to re-energize the efforts of government officials to implement the comprehensive plans that had been largely ignored during the City's fiscal crisis. The partnership model, bringing together constituencies in an alliance to promote action has had implications beyond the issue of homelessness.

The GSP differs from most of the other programs described in this issue because it constituted a new organization delivering new services. Not only did this require the hiring of new staff, but these individuals had to function in a new setting and develop a program with a mission unlike that of any other local agency. The staff needed to cope both with the pressures of a research project and the normal growth and development of a new organization. The day-to-day organization of activities has been modified on several occasions without changing the basic goals of the project. The credibility of the Hill Health Center with residents of the shelters greatly facilitated the acceptance of this new program despite its relationship to a research project operated by an institution not always trusted by many residents of the inner-city.

The evaluation of the Grant Street Partnership will provide additional information about the longer-term success of the program and help identify those men who benefit most from the type of shelter-based program described in this article. Although it is clear that a 90-day, shelter-based treatment program can have important benefits for substance abuse, the feasibility of organizing a successful shelter-based case management program serving former shelter residents in the absence of a formal continuum of residential placements still remains to be determined. Potential users constitute a heterogeneous group with motivations, strengths, and needs that vary greatly. What is clear is that shelter-based programs cannot exist in isolation if they are to succeed. What is also clear is that these programs require substantial community support if they are to survive their infancies.

REFERENCES

Spinner, G.F. & Leaf, P.J. (1992). Homelessness and drug abuse in New Haven. *Hospital and Community Psychiatry 43,* 166-168.

Sullivan, W.P., Wolk, J.L., & Hartmann, D.J. (1992). Case management in alcohol and drug treatment: Improving client outcomes. *Families in Society: The Journal of Contemporary Human Services,* 195-203.

Timney, C.B. & Graham, K. (1989). A survey of case management practices in addictions programs. *Alcoholism Treatment Quarterly 6*(3/4), 103-127.

SPECIAL POPULATIONS:
ST. LOUIS, WASHINGTON, D.C.

A Substance Abuse Recovery Program for Homeless Mothers with Children: St. Louis

Elizabeth M. Smith, PhD
Carol S. North, MD
Theresa M. Heaton, MPH

SUMMARY. Existing substance abuse programs have many limitations for homeless mothers, including the fact that they are modeled on programs for men that may not be appropriate for women. They separate mothers from their children during treatment, and they focus on adult recovery rather than being family oriented. The Grace Hill

Elizabeth M. Smith, Carol S. North, and Theresa M. Heaton are all affiliated with the Department of Psychiatry, Washington University School of Medicine, St. Louis, MO.

Address correspondence to: Elizabeth M. Smith, Washington University School of Medicine, Department of Psychiatry, 4940 Children's Place, St. Louis, MO 63110.

[Haworth co-indexing entry note]: "A Substance Abuse Recovery Program for Homeless Mothers with Children: St. Louis." Smith, Elizabeth M., Carol S. North, and Theresa M. Heaton. Co-published simultaneously in the *Alcoholism Treatment Quarterly* (The Haworth Press, Inc.) Vol. 10, No. 3/4, 1993, pp. 91-100; and: *Treatment of the Chemically Dependent Homeless: Theory and Implementation in Fourteen American Projects* (ed: Kendon J. Conrad, Cheryl I. Hultman, and John S. Lyons) The Haworth Press, Inc., 1993, pp. 91-100. Multiple copies of this article/chapter may be purchased from The Haworth Document Delivery Center [1-800-3-HAWORTH: 9:00 a.m. - 5:00 p.m. (EST)].

Family Center intervention program described in this article was designed specifically for the substance abuse treatment needs of homeless mothers in St. Louis. It blends three approaches: (1) strengthening neighbors so that they may help others, (2) traditional 12-step recovery services, and (3) Yablonsky's (1989) theory of the therapeutic community. As evidenced by a high dropout rate, this is a very difficult population to treat. Probably the most salient insight from the program to date is that creative models of service delivery are needed to reach these women and involve them in recovery programs.

INTRODUCTION

Existing substance abuse programs have many limitations for homeless families. Traditional substance abuse programs, for example, have been modeled on programs for men. They typically remove the individual from the community environment; they separate mothers from their children during treatment. The focus is more on the adult recovery process rather than on being family oriented. The threat of having a child removed, even if only temporarily, is a barrier to traditional treatment programs for homeless mothers.

Prior to the development of the current project, there were no substance abuse programs designed specifically for the needs of homeless mothers in St. Louis. This lack in services represents a significant problem in light of the increasing numbers of substance abusing homeless women. Nearly one-fourth of a random sample of 300 homeless women recently studied in St. Louis had a history of drug abuse (Smith & North, in press), more than twice the 11% lifetime rate for young women in the general population (Robins & Regier, 1991). Their 17% rate of alcohol abuse was also significantly higher than the general population rate. Overall, nearly one-third of the women had a history of substance abuse, with cocaine being the most frequently abused drug. Two-thirds of the women were mothers whose children were with them and 90% overall were mothers (Smith & North, in press). Because of these findings in St. Louis, it was apparent that a program needed to be developed to address these serious problems among this under-served population. The St. Louis homeless population reflects the current national trend towards increasing proportions of mothers among the ranks of the homeless.

This paper describes the Grace Hill Family Center intervention program which is one of three interventions developed as part of the St. Louis NIAAA demonstration project for substance abusing homeless mothers with young children. The Salvation Army based projects are described in this volume by Homan, Flick and Heaton (1993). The project described in this paper is a joint venture between Washington University School of Medicine and Grace Hill Neighborhood Services. A unique aspect of the project is the integration of settlement house and recovery philosophies in one program. Grace Hill was selected as the site for this new program for several reasons. Two of the investigators were providing mental health services to the agency's Health Services to the Homeless Program. In addition, the agency had a great deal of experience and commitment to serving low income and minority populations. Finally, with its diverse programs, Grace Hill offered the opportunity for homeless mothers who are often isolated and without social support to develop relationships and a sense of belonging to the neighborhood's community.

GRACE HILL BACKGROUND

Prior to the current program, Grace Hill lacked a substance abuse program, but it did have considerable experience in serving populations with high rates of these problems. In addition, it had previously operated an emergency shelter for homeless women. Grace Hill's mission was rooted in the settlement house philosophy of helping neighbors to help themselves and each other, for example, by hiring neighborhood residents. The agency had a long history as a multi-service social service agency dating back to the early part of the 1900s. Its diverse programs included a comprehensive health center, housing, child daycare, educational programs, job placement, and other services to support neighborhood residents.

The initial plan was to locate the program in a multi-family building in the neighborhood. The "NIMBY" ("Not in My Back Yard") phenomenon made this difficult. Instead it was decided to operate the program in the building that formerly housed the Grace Hill emergency shelter for women and children. To avoid confusion with the old shelter and to avoid stigmatizing the women in relation to a "drug center," the name Grace Hill Family Center was chosen. The initial purpose of the program was to provide substance-free, supportive housing to women in recovery. The model for the program was that of a modified therapeutic community.

THE INTERVENTION MODEL

This new intervention is based on the belief that recovery is possible when clients seeking sobriety help each other. The model is a blend of three approaches: (1) Grace Hill's settlement house philosophy of strengthening neighbors so that neighbors help one another; (2) traditional recovery services which draw on the 12-step approach in the context of group therapy; and (3) Yablonsky's (1989) theory of the therapeutic community in which addicts act as co-therapists.

The model which emerges is a modified therapeutic community, supported by professional recovery staff and programming, external 12-step groups, and Grace Hill neighbors and peers. It diverges from the true therapeutic community model in the following ways: no detoxification is provided; the range of therapeutic modalities is restricted; the majority of the staff are not in recovery themselves; and there are fewer opportunities for employment within the center, although these opportunities exist within the larger Grace Hill system. The goals of the Grace Hill Family Center are the promotion of recovery of homeless families with chemical dependency, stabilization of the family unit, movement toward economic self-sufficiency, and housing stabilization.

This study is attempting to determine how most efficiently and economically these goals can be met. To do so, it compares the outcomes of women randomized to the residential group (i.e., those living at the Family Center) to those of women who attend only during the day and live elsewhere during the first phase of the program. During this time, both groups receive the same daily recovery and neighborhood services; the difference is that some are settled in a stable residence and others stay in precarious, temporary living spaces.

PRELIMINARY FINDINGS

Women are eligible for the program if they are homeless or in imminent danger of homelessness, have a past or current problem with substance abuse, have one or more children ages 12 or younger in their care, are nonviolent, nonpsychotic, and not actively suicidal. Referral sources include shelters, treatment programs and social service agencies. However, nearly half the women are referred through the Grace Hill neighborhood system and neighbors themselves.

The Center houses seven families. It also holds the program's meeting space, child care space, kitchen and dining room, and offices for staff. Women and their children attend the program daily. All children receive child care while their mothers participate in program activities; those in the residential group live with their mothers at the Center.

In the first 16 months of operation, 87 women have been referred to the program. They range in age from 20 to 46 years; the average age is 30. Essentially all of the clients are black. Sixty-two percent of the women are single, never married; 37% are separated or divorced; and 1% are widowed. Nearly half of the women (49%) do not have a high school diploma or GED; the mean number of years of education is 11.5. These women have a total of 299 children. The range was between 1 and 8 children; the mean was 3.7. Children ranged in age from ages of 1 month to 26 years; mean age was 7.4 years.

The majority (76%) of the women reported current cocaine abuse and 30% reported both cocaine and alcohol abuse. Eight percent met criteria only for a current diagnosis of alcohol abuse. Two-thirds of the women reported prior treatment for chemical dependency problems; they had been in treatment between 1 and 6 times (the mean = 2).

Seventeen percent of the women who were accepted did not enter the program. Approximately one-fourth of the women have completed, or are still in, the program. Another 41% left prematurely (against staff advice) and 17% were asked to leave the program because they violated house rules.

DESCRIPTION OF THE PROGRAM

The program, which lasts one year, has two phases. Phase I is centered around a treatment/recovery model. It is a substance-free, 90-day *therapeutic community* setting for 14 female-headed homeless families with children under age 12. Entry into the program is voluntary, implying that some level of motivation and commitment to become substance free must exist, even though the motives may not necessarily be pure.

Treatment consists of a basic 12-step approach that involves recovering women as co-therapists in a supportive group environment (Yablonsky, 1989). The recovery intervention in Phase I is accomplished in both group and individual treatment modalities.

The key component of the therapeutic community is a family orientation that provides structure and direction to the recovering woman who needs external structure during this phase. This structure nurtures the sharing of emotional experiences that allows the recovering mother to feel accepted and want to stay. An initial period of separation from past, frequently unhealthy, relationships facilitates bonding into this new family. Attention is then directed toward treating the woman's relationships and she can begin to think about how she will relate to a partner or other family member who may be part of her problem. Within this therapeutic community structure someone is always available with whom the recovering woman can discuss her real and immediate problems. These informal talks provide invaluable spontaneous nurturance of her desire to resolve important issues in her life.

Neighborhood based stabilization and supportive services are offered by Grace Hill neighbors beginning in Phase I and include the Member Organized Resource Exchange (M.O.R.E.) system, the neighborhood college, and careers center as well as access to health care. This system offers specific courses in which residents participate along with other neighborhood women.

All those living in the residence are required to pay a percentage of their AFDC benefits for rent and to set up and maintain a savings account. Although the duration of the first phase of the program is approximately three months, some women may stay as long as six months. Flexibility allows women to progress at their own pace, as not all will be ready to move into housing after three months.

Upon graduation from Phase I, the client lives and works in the community with less structure, maintaining affiliation with the therapeutic community to which she was bonded during Phase I. Phase II provides ongoing professionally facilitated support group participation as well as regular assessment and individual counseling by a trained, culturally sensitive professional with special focus on relapse prevention. After 30 days in Phase II the client earns the privilege of joining the alumnae group, an affiliation which can continue long after completing the program. Clients meet together in regular planned, structured events to continually refresh and revitalize their therapeutic community bond and to further reduce their vulnerability to relapse during the precarious first few months after graduation from Phase I.

In Phase II clients also receive regular stabilization home visits from both the aftercare case manager as well as trained peer counselors who work with carefully coordinated efforts to enable the client and her family to maintain stable housing, income, entitlements, and resources.

IMPLEMENTATION ISSUES

As might be expected in developing a new program, implementation of the model can never go as smoothly as designing it. Much of the first year has been spent dealing with various implementation issues. The two most crucial implementation issues were recruitment and retention.

At the start of the program it was decided to fill the residence first so that the therapeutic community could be built rapidly. Once the residential slots were filled, assignments were randomized. During the informed consent procedure clients were told there was a 50/50 chance of getting into one group or another–like a lottery. When the first seven referrals all received residential assignment, referral sources were pleased that their clients had a place to stay. As nonresidential assignments were made, however, clients and their referral sources were increasingly disappointed. Upon receiving assignment to the (nonresidential) day group, many failed to show up for the program and others soon dropped out. Once referral sources learned there was no guaranteed residential placement at any time, referrals slowed. Despite efforts to work out relationships between Grace Hill Family Center and temporary shelters to arrange housing for those in the day group, the randomization process, so important to the research design, remains a threat to the program itself.

Despite recovery-specific recruitment efforts, the chief incentive for entering the program remains the hope of getting housing–in much the same way that the fear of losing a job or spouse motivates their middle class counterparts. The program recognizes this reality and deals with it directly in the intake process by describing in honest detail the elements of the program and its emphasis on recovery. Prospective clients are informed that help with housing is part of the program–but only when about 90 days of sobriety have been achieved.

Another challenge to recruitment was the failure to act immediately upon inquiries. Many of these were from addicted women calling in a brief moment of sobriety or from a pay phone or from a shelter. Many referrals were lost either because staff did not reach them or because the motivation to seek treatment did not last long enough. To address this problem, the intake procedure was streamlined. Two intake workers rather than one handled calls immediately as they came in and arranged for an eligibility screening within 24-48 hours.

In addition to this internal change, the rest of the staff was given inservice training to help them recognize the role they play in promoting effective recruitment. Now they also help ensure that prospective clients make it to their eligibility screening. For example, whenever possible the evening staff makes reminder calls the night before a screening and double-checks on a client's need for transportation and/or childcare for the screening. All staff welcome the prospective client upon her arrival, help her and her children get comfortable, and encourage them to stay for program activities once the screening is completed. These interventions are aimed at engaging the client enough for her to choose to return and start the program because her initial contact was so positive and attractive.

Currently the project is working to strengthen and expand its referral base within the greater social service community through the distribution of a program fact sheet and follow-up calls to homeless, outreach, and treatment programs in the area. Similar efforts are targeting services, programs, and departments within the Grace Hill system. Within the approach there is acknowledgement of the difficulty agencies face when their client needs shelter as well as treatment. But agencies are also helped to understand the program's commitment to finding temporary shelter for the clients as well as permanent housing later on in their recovery journey.

As the recruitment challenges were dealt with, client retention issues also developed. The drop-out rate was high in the early months of the program. Client retention is directly related to the level of motivation and commitment to recovery that clients experience. Recognizing that this motivation is often weak and diffuse and related to housing, a specific orientation process was developed wherein the client would be assessed and interviewed comprehensively in her first week. It was hoped that this process would help the client come to a deeper awareness of her need for treatment and lead to greater commitment. Detailed substance abuse, health, and mental health evaluations; parenting and educational assessments; and in-depth program orientation were provided.

About a year into the program, the daily schedule was changed for the client's first 30 days in order to strengthen the treatment approach and, consequently, to enhance client motivation. The changes limited new clients to program activities which focus most on recovery. After 30 days, clients could broaden their perspectives and begin to explore education/ employment options, spend more time in parenting classes, and do groundwork for housing placements as they kept working at recovery.

Day group retention has continued to be an ongoing problem for the project. The turnover is rapid and high–so much so that the nonresidential group never stays full. Precarious housing arrangements, ongoing family obligations, manipulations and crises of the extended family, transportation problems, and continued exposure to drugs make it difficult for the nonresidential group members to maintain their involvement in the program.

Although staff have worked to strengthen the program's relationship with shelters in the city, they still face a challenge every time a client is assigned to nonresidential status. Unless the client can be placed in a shelter that very day, chances are the client will not participate. Homeless women are not placed in city shelters unless they have absolutely nowhere else to go–regardless of whether the placement will facilitate participation in the program. Over time, the staff members are becoming more effective dealing with the nuances of shelter placement.

Some nonresidential clients simply refuse to consider placement in a shelter and remain doubled up with a relative or friend. Their attendance at the day program may be sporadic, and clients present many good excuses for missing program days. It is difficult to determine what excuses are genuine and which are addiction-related. The program has developed a communication system for nonresidential clients. Calls are made if the client has not contacted the Center. If no telephone contact is made, a home visit is attempted so that the client's situation can be assessed and she can be encouraged to rejoin the group of women who fight for their sobriety.

Another major retention issue is related to staff effectiveness. Because the Grace Hill settlement house philosophy rests on the conviction that neighbors are best suited to help neighbors, the Grace Hill Family Center staff is made up largely of paraprofessional neighbors. Few of the staff had been introduced to substance abuse treatment practices when this project started; two of the four professionals on staff had specialized substance abuse training. Even with inservice training, it was a challenge for the staff to both learn and act on principles that seemed to conflict with their natural inclination to trust and help clients directly (i.e., co-dependent or naive helping behaviors). Clients themselves identified the problem they faced in their recovery when they could outwit the staff–a problem that contributed to the retention problem.

Chemical dependency education and specific skills training for the staff have been implemented. Ongoing feedback and processing of client interactions and incidents help the staff to deal more consistently and effectively with the clients. As the competency level in the specific area of recovery support continues to grow, the retention issue should diminish.

In future projects with agencies that have never provided recovery services, it is recommended that intensive staff training be initiated before clients are ever accepted. Secondly, weekly debriefings should be scheduled to ensure quality processing time once clients have been accepted into the program. Finally, it is important to ask the clients regularly for their feedback and suggestions for making the services more consistent, reliable, and effective.

CONCLUSIONS

This project which was designed to meet the needs of homeless mothers with substance abuse problems is providing valuable insights into the needs of this special population. Probably the most salient insight is that creative models of service delivery are needed to reach these women and involve them in recovery programs. As evidenced by the high dropout rate, this is a difficult population to treat. Exploration of factors associated with positive outcomes among women successfully completing the program should provide valuable guidance for the future.

AUTHOR'S NOTE

This project is supported by National Institute on Alcohol Abuse and Alcoholism Grant AA08335.

The authors acknowledge the contributions from Grace Hill Neighborhood Services of Mr. Richard Gram, Executive Director, Ms. Betty Marver, MSW, Managing Director, and Ms. Nancy Owens, Director of Community Health, in developing this cooperative effort, and thank the staff and women who have contributed to its ongoing progress.

REFERENCES

Homan, S.M., Flick, L.H., Heaton, T.H., Mayer, J.P., & Klein, M. (in press). Reaching beyond crisis management: Design and implementation of extended shelter-based services for chemically dependent homeless women and their children. *Alcoholism Treatment Quarterly.*

Robins L.N. & Regier D.A. (1991). *Psychiatric Disorders in America: The Epidemiologic Catchment Area Study.* New York: The Free Press.

Smith, E.M., North, C.S. & Spitznagel, E.L. (in press). Alcohol, drugs, and psychiatric comorbidity among homeless women: An epidemiologic study. *Journal of Clinical Psychiatry.*

Yablonsky, L. (1989). *The Therapeutic Community: A Successful Approach for Treating Substance Abusers.* New York: Gardner Press.

Reaching Beyond Crisis Management: Design and Implementation of Extended Shelter-Based Services for Chemically Dependent Homeless Women and Their Children: St. Louis

Sharon M. Homan, PhD
Louise H. Flick, MSN, Dr PH
Theresa M. Heaton, BSN, MPH
Jeffrey P. Mayer, PhD
Michael Klein, ACSW

SUMMARY. A rapidly increasing share of the homeless population consists of substance-abusing mothers and their children. Traditional

Sharon M. Homan is Associate Professor of Biostatistics, Department of Community Health, School of Public Health, St. Louis University, 3663 Lindell Blvd., St. Louis, MO 63108-3342. Louise H. Flick is Associate Professor, School of Nursing, St. Louis University, 3525 Caroline Street, St. Louis, MO 63104. Theresa M. Heaton is Project Director, 'Families with a Future,' Department of Psychiatry, School of Medicine, Washington University, 4949 Audubon, St. Louis, MO 63110. Jeffrey P. Mayer is Assistant Professor, Department of Community Health, School of Public Health, St. Louis University, 3663 Lindell Blvd., St. Louis, MO 63108-3342. Michael Klein is Divisional Director of Social Services, The Salvation Army, Midland Division, 3800 Lindell Blvd., St. Louis, MO 63108.

[Haworth co-indexing entry note]: "Reaching Beyond Crisis Management: Design and Implementation of Extended Shelter-Based Services for Chemically Dependent Homeless Women and Their Children: St. Louis." Homan, Sharon M. et al. Co-published simultaneously in the *Alcoholism Treatment Quarterly* (The Haworth Press, Inc.) Vol. 10, No. 3/4, 1993, pp. 101-112; and: *Treatment of the Chemically Dependent Homeless: Theory and Implementation in Fourteen American Projects* (ed: Kendon J. Conrad, Cheryl I. Hultman, and John S. Lyons) The Haworth Press, Inc., 1993, pp. 101-112. Multiple copies of this article/chapter may be purchased from The Haworth Document Delivery Center [1-800-3-HAWORTH: 9:00 a.m. - 5:00 p.m. (EST)].

101

family shelter programs have employed a crisis management approach addressing only short-term and immediate concerns. The St. Louis "Families with a Future" research demonstration project extends and enhances traditional 60-day shelter services with twelve months of case management and/or comprehensive family and child development support services. This paper describes the setting and target group, presents the extended interventions and their theoretical basis, and discusses development of the researcher-clinician coalition responsible for project implementation.

The St. Louis *Families with a Future* research demonstration project is designed to examine the effectiveness of three interventions which address the special needs of homeless substance-abusing women with children. One of these interventions, the modified therapeutic community at Grace Hill, is described in this issue by Smith, North, and Heaton (1992). The other two interventions have been initiated at two Salvation Army family shelters. The Grace Hill program offers substance abuse treatment and recovery in a 90-day therapeutic community setting for up to 14 mothers and their children. The Grace Hill program directly recruits homeless women with active substance abuse problems. The Salvation Army, on the other hand, receives clients into their two family shelters who are referred because of their immediate need for shelter. The Salvation Army interventions are aimed at helping the mothers recognize and manage their substance abuse problems, linking these women with treatment programs and housing opportunities, and actively engaging each mother and her children through a personal relationship with the case manager.

The purpose of this paper is twofold: to describe the Salvation Army-based project (the target population and sample, the objectives and theoretical basis for the interventions, and the evaluation research); and to identify key implementation issues. In particular, we focus on the challenges and successes in building and fostering a strong team of professionals to implement these interventions.

BACKGROUND

As Smith et al. (1992) have summarized, homeless families are a rapidly growing subgroup nationally and locally. The Center on Budget and Policy Priorities concluded that "Although the affordable housing crisis is national in scope, it is particularly acute in St. Louis" (Allen and Lazere, 1992). St. Louis has the highest percent of people who pay more than 30% of their income on housing. The major problems are lack of affordable housing, physically deficient housing, and overcrowding. Such problems force many poor families to move from shelter to shelter with brief stays with extended family. If housing is located, it is typically substandard and inadequate.

The Salvation Army family shelters, like most shelters in the St. Louis area, are faced with a steady stream of clients and long referral lists. The clients who enter the family shelters are predominantly African-American women (95-97%) with young children. Many of these families have multiple social problems, economic and educational problems, as well as, substance abuse disorders. In the last three years the estimated prevalence of chemical dependency among mothers in the two Salvation Army shelters has increased from about 10% in 1989 to 40% in 1991. In our study sample, crack cocaine (70%) and alcohol (12%) are the primary problem drugs. The growing rate of substance abuse among residents has strained the services and resources of the Salvation Army shelters.

The demonstration project sites are the Salvation Army family shelters: Family Haven (FH) in St. Louis City, and Community in Partnership (CIP) in St. Louis County. Both shelters are quite similar in philosophy, resources, staff, clients, and services provided. Both provide up to 60 days of shelter and needed services to homeless families. These services include case management, child care, daily living skills development and education (e.g., parenting and money management classes). Most often, the focus of services is on crisis management, that is, attending to the client's immediate needs for housing assistance, linking with the school system, securing entitlements, substance abuse treatment, and assistance with child custody. Given the unfortunate combination of many problems and limited program sources, it is difficult for the mothers and shelter staff to look beyond these emergency needs. Yet, even when there is opportunity to apply the full set of available services during their shelter stay, most families need intensive ongoing post-shelter support, particularly families with substance abuse problems. These families are not prepared to 'make it on their own' when they leave the shelter.

BRIDGING THE GAPS

In 1990, our research team from St. Louis University joined as partners with the Salvation Army to initiate a proposal to the National Institute on Alcohol Abuse and Alcoholism (NIAAA). Prior to proposal submission, the research team met frequently with staff from several local service agencies to: (1) understand the issues of service delivery to homeless families with chemical dependency and addiction; (2) gain support and credibility both with the Salvation Army as well as with other community agencies; and (3) create a sense of mutuality with the Salvation Army in the determination of the intervention strategies, their implementation, and the research protocol. These purposes were largely achieved as a result of the high value placed on research by the Salvation Army's Director of Social Services, the long history of the Salvation Army working with alcoholic clients, the open-mindedness of the shelter administrators to explore new strategies to provide services, the research team's genuine commitment to homeless clients as persons versus research subjects, and a willingness of the research team to understand the agency's history, philosophy, and mission.

During the several months that we worked with Salvation Army agency staff to initiate our proposal, we became increasingly aware of the gaps in the existing system of services to homeless families, particularly those for chemically dependent mothers. In the 1980s, the local Salvation Army developed a strategy (the Homeless Continuum Model, HCM; Hutchinson, 1981) to provide homeless families with a continuum of services aimed at moving families through progressive service stages: stabilization (usually 60 days in emergency shelter); relocation to transitional housing; permanent housing and community reintegration. The existing shelter services were considered inadequate, however, for the growing number of families with substance abuse problems, particularly for supportive services to motivate and sustain client participation in substance abuse treatment and aftercare. In particular, two major gaps in the continuum model were identified. First, clients move in and out of treatment and service agencies with no systematic follow-up or consistent relationship with a provider. Secondly, comprehensive family services are needed to engage families, support recovery, and promote healthy individual and family functioning.

To address these gaps in the HCM for homeless mothers and their families, we proposed two intervention strategies: (1) extension of case management from 60 days in shelter to 12 months post-shelter entry; and (2) enhancement and extension of family services to 12 months post-shelter entry. The family services component, called Building Blocks, was enhanced through the addition of a family therapist to the team of child development specialists already working at the St. Louis County shelter, CIP.

INTERVENTION DESIGN AND THEORETICAL BASIS

The target population consists of homeless women with child(ren) who enter the shelter system in the St. Louis area. To be eligible for the study, the client must be referred to FH or CIP, and have past or current substance abuse or dependency. The projected sample size is approximately 60 women (and 150 children) to be enrolled at each of the two shelters over a two year period.

Upon meeting study eligibility criteria, clients are administered the baseline interview battery. At both FH and CIP, clients are then randomly assigned to either the customary 60-day case management services (50%) or the extended case management services (50%). All clients at CIP receive the enhanced Building Blocks services which are not available at FH. In summary, the design is a partially randomized 2 by 2 factorial experiment for which approximately 30 families are enrolled into each of four groups: (1) customary case management with no Building Blocks intervention (FH); (2) extended case management with no Building Block intervention (FH); (3) customary case management with Building Blocks (CIP); and (4) extended case management with Building Blocks (CIP). This design permits us to examine the efficacy of each factor (i.e., intervention) as well as the interaction effect of the two interventions. Evaluation of this experiment includes both process (e.g., service delivery and implementation) and outcome evaluation. A comprehensive battery of structured interviews is conducted on each client and her children. Data are gathered at study entry, and at 6, 12, and 18 months after baseline. Extensive semi-structured interviews have been collected on a subsample of 12 participants to gain an understanding of the mothers' epistemologies and their communication strategies with their case managers and their children.

The extended and enhanced interventions are designed to promote client engagement and participation in goal setting; move the agency and staff toward an approach to clients of empowerment and mutuality; and directly address substance abuse problems of the mother in the context of the nuclear and extended families. Before describing these two interventions, it is helpful to further describe the women and children receiving these services: 61% of the mothers were never married (96% single); families have between 1 and 9 children (65% have 3 or more children); 55% of the mothers report being physically abused by their husband or partner; and the families have been homeless on average for 12 months. In the month prior to entering shelter, the women received an average of $209 in AFDC and $195 in foodstamps yet spent an average of $96 (up to $800) on drugs and alcohol. Many of the children suffer developmental delays and have very disrupted school and family lives.

Building Blocks

The goal of the Building Blocks intervention is to address family dysfunction through child development services and family therapy. The child development specialists use a three-prong approach of assessment, treatment, and advocacy. The educational and developmental problems of the children in the family are assessed, and individualized learning plans are developed to guide the mother (fathers and teachers, when possible) in promoting knowledge and skill development and managing child behavior. To become an active partner in the development of her children, the mother needs to assume a parental role of nurturer and caregiver. Frequently, however, homeless substance-abusing mothers have a sense of powerlessness and are unable to perform their roles. Systems theory guided family therapy seeks to change the family system by modifying interactions within the family, as well as interactions of the family in the broader social community. As a mother moves into her addiction, she models more childlike behavior and the family system becomes inverted, that is, the mother effectively becomes a 'child' thereby abdicating her parental role. The family therapist becomes part of that family system and helps the family build a better functioning system. This empowers the mother (or parents) to model a more healthy parental role which serves to reinforce the mother's partnership with the developmental specialist and teachers in her children's education and development.

As an adjunct to systems-based family therapy, Building Blocks also includes individual and group therapy based on the 12-step program to support client recovery. The therapist is an African-American master's trained psychologist with considerable experience working with chemically dependent families. She expresses cultural sensitivity and has a high level of competence in assessing African-American families, recognizing the diversity of family structures and processes, and the importance of the extended family (Logan, 1990).

Extended Case Management

The extended case management intervention is staffed by an all female racially mixed team of public health nurses (PHNs) and social workers (MSWs). We selected a team of PHNs and MSWs to meet the special needs of homeless women in their childbearing years with very young children. The majority of the children are under five years of age and experience high rates of behavioral, developmental, and medical problems. Each case manager has a primary caseload of 6-10 families. The case managers meet regularly, with other team members for case conferences, mutual support and training. At times a case manager may call upon another team member to provide direct service to one of her clients. This modified team approach (Reineke and Greenley, 1986) allows the development of individual long-term client relationships even as the team shares responsibility for all cases, hence benefiting from the multidisciplinary perspective and expertise of the team. This team approach emphasizes resource and service linkage to meet basic needs (enablement), facilitating the client's ability to define goals (empowerment), and building on existing family strengths (enhancement) (Wasik, Bryant, and Lyons, 1990; Johnson and Rubin, 1983). After a client leaves the shelter, the case manager actively initiates weekly to monthly face-to-face contact. Unlike most of the shelter-based case managers, the extended case management team has experience and training in addiction etiology, assessment and intervention.

Key to the success of both long-term interventions is continued client engagement post-shelter. The client's willingness to continue with the case manager is threatened by many circumstances: abusive family situations, drug use, difficulty engaging significant others (e.g., client's boyfriend or mother), or client's feeling threatened by case manager.

Case management practice has been structured on Antonovsky's Salu-togenesis Model. Sense of coherence (SOC), the central concept of this theory, is a "global orientation that expresses the extent to which one has a pervasive enduring, though dynamic, feeling of confidence that (1) the stimuli deriving from one's internal and external environments . . . are explicable [comprehensibility]; (2) the resources are available to one to meet the demands . . . [manageability]; and (3) these demands are worthy of investment and engagement [meaningfulness]" (Antonovsky, 1987). The theory posits that progress on the three dimensions leads to greater SOC, and therefore improved coping with extreme adversity. The SOC dimensions (comprehensibility, manageability and meaningfulness) are a useful guide for setting priorities with clients, structuring case manage-ment activities, and developing positive cognitions and attitudes that lead to empowering clients to deal actively with the problems confronting them. For example, progress on the meaningfulness dimension is reflected in the client's choice to continue to stay in treatment so she doesn't lose custody of her children.

The SOC theory was not chosen to dictate case management practice; rather a praxis approach has been taken. Praxis is the lived and living engagement of theory and action. Rather than a static movement from theory to practice, and thereby creating a disjuncture between the two, a praxis approach allows practice to generate and refine theory in a dynamic process. A dialectic has been created such that the team members put the SOC concepts into action, come together and reflect on their experience, and then refine their understanding and action. This process has given the team a common basis for praxis and has invited them into ongoing dialogue. This dialogue has fostered a strong sense of collegiality and has been an important element in team building.

IMPLEMENTATION ISSUES AND TEAM BUILDING

Implementation of our interventions has required us to address a number of issues: team building; client engagement and retention; the salary structures for professionals in the community and at the FH and CIP shelters; systematic record keeping and data collection at the agencies (provider-level data); networking with treatment agencies; client referrals into shelter; staff training, particularly in areas related to addiction; as well as issues related to racial consciousness and cultural sensitivity. In this section we focus on one of these implementation issues: team building and development. In particular, we discuss the role of research and service professionals in the project and our efforts to develop a truly collaborative relationship among researchers and agency managers and providers.

A key to our building and developing a strong research-service coalition has been the role of the project director. The project director facilitates the implementation of the interventions (including ongoing staff supervision, training and development), manages the research interviewers and data collection personnel, and helps ensure the integrity of the research protocol (e.g., randomization, client recruitment and retention, and confidentiality). The project director also networks with local homeless providers and substance abuse agencies. Thus, she is a liaison between agencies, providers, and the research team, helping us keep a common mission of promoting compassionate and effective delivery of services to homeless mothers and their families. Also critical to our sustaining an effective research-clinical coalition is the regular communication between the investigators and the shelter administrators and staff. The investigators are readily available to meet with agency staff to address budget considerations, participate in staff recruitment and hiring, and to discuss strategies and policies for client engagement, management, and retention.

A challenge to team building was the integration of the new providers into the existing shelter staff. Mutual supervision of the new staff by the appropriate shelter supervisor and by the project director has been effective. The project team provided specialized orientation and training to meet the mutual research and agency goal of forming a cohesive, effective intervention team, which can be integrated into the existing team of usual services providers at each site. The orientation objectives included learning the agency culture and the intricacies of shelter casework; exploring the theoretical model underlying intervention practice–and actually contributing to its development and application (i.e., praxis); becoming familiar with community resources and building essential community networks; and, developing expertise in addictions.

Ongoing training continues to help meet these objectives. The intervention case management team, family therapist, project director, and investigator meet weekly to discuss clients, intervention strategies, community resources, housing, confrontation and other issues around chemical dependency, as well as to dialogue about the SOC model and its underlying principles and implications.

Of primary importance to case management team and Building Blocks team development is ongoing education and training in the etiology, treatment, and management of substance abuse and addiction. The professional and support staff at FH and CIP had minimal training or experience with substance abusers. Therefore, we developed two training series (20 sessions) on substance abuse for all Salvation Army staff (including the case managers, family therapist, child development specialists, the night aids, janitors, and secretaries) as well as staff at the Grace Hill project site (see Smith et al., 1992) and from other agencies in the Homeless Services Network. These well-attended series stimulated dialogue, raised challenges to the current system, and gave staff an opportunity to express their frustrations. Topics included relapse prevention, parenting drug-affected children, cultural sensitivity, women's issues in recovery, effective case management strategies with chemically dependent clients.

PRELIMINARY FINDINGS AND RECOMMENDATIONS

In summary, the researchers, in partnership with the Salvation Army, designed and implemented interventions to meet the needs of chemically dependent homeless mothers by expanding and enhancing services beyond crisis management. While we are only at the half-way point of client enrollment, thus precluding unbiased statistical description and analysis of the data, we can discuss our preliminary findings with regard to implementation issues and client perceptions.

An important finding is that the NIAAA demonstration project has increased the Salvation Army's attention and resources to service delivery to substance abusing mothers and families. A greater proportion of clientele with substance abuse continues to bring resolve to FH and CIP administrators to deal directly with a problem with which many shelters choose not to cope by refusing entry to clients with drug use problems. Since the project's inception, CIP has begun developing resources to become one of the State's Medicaid-funded outpatient Comprehensive Substance Treatment and Rehabilitation (CSTAR) sites.

A second finding is that the case management team continues to develop positively in their interactions with clients and one another. A sense of mutual trust has developed among the team members. It is common for them at case conferences to appraise their practice honestly and to recognize times when personal issues interfere with practice. Frank and open discussion of interventions occurs. The case managers have voiced how important the informal support of one another is, particularly in reducing the stress associated with client termination or refusal of further intervention.

Finally, we've learned much from extensive (8+ hours per client) taped encounters with a subsample of 12 clients. We examined the epistemologic development of these women using the methods developed by Belenky and colleagues (Belenky, Clinchy, Goldberger, and Tarule, 1986; Bond and Belenky, 1991) to understand women's ways of knowing and women's experience in gaining a voice. Our study has provided a means for understanding the *way* services are to be presented if the clients are to access treatment programs and other services. Many of the women see experience as their primary means of validating knowledge and that the only way a person can really know something is to have also experienced it. Group therapy, facilitated by the family therapist, gives these clients an opportunity to belong to a supportive group in which they can express themselves and gain from the experience of the other women. The extended case management intervention with its approach of mutuality, and what one case manager called 'sisterhood', works to break down authoritative barriers, giving clients a voice in their lives and a safer opportunity for growth.

A third point is the importance of anticipating the disequilibrium that occurs in a social service agency when the agency adopts a new focus on substance abuse and accepts increased numbers of chemically dependent mothers and children. Many of the existing shelter policies, staffing, orientation to clients, and implementation of regulations are likely to be challenged. Further, in these family shelters where substance abuse treatment is not provided, yet chemically dependent families are served, staff training is essential to avoid having staff working at cross purposes. We found inservices and training useful for all levels of staff (including program aides and janitors). Finally, an interdisciplinary team with varied approaches enriches team development and individual practice. The praxis approach has been successful in improving practice and refining theory.

Implementation of the extended case management and Building Blocks interventions at two Salvation Army family shelters in St. Louis has significantly impacted the agency in terms of its future service delivery to homeless families with substance abuse problems. The agency has sought to better understand and deliver services which directly facilitate substance abuse treatment and recovery; and, is seeking opportunities to expand transitional housing availability. On the other hand, the external environment continues to worsen locally. Shelter waiting lists for homeless families are growing. Social service agency resources have declined as has the availability of inpatient treatment for chemical dependency through Medicaid reimbursement, and most significantly, the availability of transitional and permanent housing for the poor. While the proposed interventions show promise, without improvements in housing availability and access to treatment, the interventions cannot succeed.

AUTHOR'S NOTE

This Research is currently supported by the National Institute on Alcohol Abuse and Alcoholism (U01 AA08804-02) under the Cooperative Agreements for Research Demonstration Projects on Alcohol and Other Drug Abuse Treatment for Homeless Persons.

Our special thanks to Krystal Lisle, MSW, Director of Family Haven, and Doug Eller, MSW, Director of Community in Partnership, and to the many Salvation Army Staff who have cooperated in this joint venture.

REFERENCES

Allen, C. and Lazere, E.B. (1992). *St. Louis Missouri. A place to call home. The crisis in housing for the poor.* Washington D.C.: Center on Budget and Policy Priorities.

Antonovsky, A. (1987). *Unraveling the mystery of health.* San Francisco: Jossey-Bass Publishers.

Belenky, M.F., Clinchy, B.M., Goldberger, N.R. and Tarule, J.M. (1986). *Women's ways of knowing: The development of self, voice, and mind.* New York: Basic Books.

Freeman, E.M. (1990). *The addiction process: effective social work approaches.* New York: Longman Publishers.

Harvey, M.R. and D'Ercole, A. (1990). The process of designing and implementing programs for homeless families. In E.L. Bassuk, R.W. Carman and L.F. Weinreb (Eds.), *Community care for homeless families: A program design manual* (pp. 17-24). Washington, D.C.: Interagency Council on Homelessness.

Hutchison, W.J., Stretch, J., Anderman, S. et al. (1981). *A profile of the emergency housing program in the City of St. Louis.* A joint demonstration project of the Community Development Agency and the Salvation Army, St. Louis, MO.

Johnson, P. and Rubin, A. (1983). Case management in mental health: A Social work domain? *Social Work,* 1, pp. 49-55.

Linsalata, P. and Novak, T. (1991, December 11). KC gets less U.S. money, builds more housing. *St. Louis Post-Dispatch*, p. 18a.

Logan, S.M.L., Freeman, E.M. and McRoy, R.G. (1990). *Social work practice with black families: A culturally specific perspective.* New York: Longman Publishers.

National Institute on Alcohol Abuse and Alcoholism (1991). *Application of case management in alcohol and drug dependence: Matching techniques and populations.* (DHHS Publication No. ADM 91-1766). Washington, D.C.: U.S. Government Printing Offices.

Novak, T., and Linsalata, P. (1991, December 8). Opportunity denied: St. Louis uses the poor to aid wealthier neighborhoods. *St. Louis Post-Dispatch*, pp. 1, 13, 15.

Reineke, B. and Greenley, J. R. (1986). Organizational analysis of three community support program models. *Hospital and Community Psychiatry, 37,* 634-639.

Schilling R., Schinke, S. and Weatherly, R. (1988). Service trends in a conservative era: Social workers rediscover the past. *Social Work, 43*(1), 5-9.

Smith, E.M., North C., and Heaton, T.M. (in press). A substance abuse recovery program for homeless mothers with children. *Alcoholism Treatment Quarterly,* 10(3/4).

Wasik, B., Bryant, D. and Lyons, M. (1990). *Home visiting: Procedures for helping families.* Newbury Park, California: Sage Publications.

Process Evaluation
in the Washington, D.C.,
Dual Diagnosis Project

Robert E. Drake, MD, PhD
Richard R. Bebout, PhD
Ernest Quimby, PhD
Gregory B. Teague, PhD
Maxine Harris, PhD
Jeff P. Roach, PhD

SUMMARY. In health service demonstration research, process evaluation refers to measuring the program itself rather than its effects. A model-guided process evaluation includes specifying the treatment model, assessing its implementation, monitoring the fidelity of the model throughout the project, assessing model exposure and absorption, and helping to understand the program's intermediate effects

Robert Drake and Gregory Teague are affiliated with the New Hampshire-Dartmouth Psychiatric Research Center, 105 Pleasant Street, Concord, NH; Richard Bebout and Maxine Harris are affiliated with Community Connections, 1512 Pennsylvania Ave., S.E., Washington, D.C.; Ernest Quimby is affiliated with Howard University, P.O. Box 987, Washington, D.C.; and Jeff Roach was formerly with Community Connections.

Address correspondence to: Robert Drake, New Hampshire-Dartmouth Psychiatric Research Center, 2 Whipple Place, Lebanon, NH 03766.

This article was supported by U.S. Public Health Service Grants U01-AA-08840 from the National Institute on Alcohol Abuse and Alcoholism and K02-MH-00839 from the National Institute of Mental Health.

[Haworth co-indexing entry note]: "Process Evaluation in the Washington, D.C., Dual Diagnosis Project." Drake, Robert E. et al. Co-published simultaneously in the *Alcoholism Treatment Quarterly* (The Haworth Press, Inc.) Vol. 10, No. 3/4, 1993, pp. 113-124; and: *Treatment of the Chemically Dependent Homeless: Theory and Implementation in Fourteen American Projects* (ed: Kendon J. Conrad, Cheryl I. Hultman, and John S. Lyons) The Haworth Press, Inc., 1993, pp. 113-124. Multiple copies of this article/chapter may be purchased from The Haworth Document Delivery Center [1-800-3-HAWORTH: 9:00 a.m. - 5:00 p.m. (EST)].

(i.e., proximal outcomes) as well as final effects (i.e., distal outcomes). To illustrate the mechanisms and uses of a process evaluation, this article describes the Washington, D.C., Dual Diagnosis Project, a research demonstration project for homeless persons with co-occurring severe mental disorders and substance use disorders.

Among the population of homeless persons, those who are dually diagnosed with both severe mental disorder and substance use disorder comprise a subgroup with multiple, interacting impairments and special needs (Drake, Osher, and Wallach, 1991; Minkoff and Drake, 1992). Addressing their needs is complicated by fragmentation of the formal service delivery system (Minkoff and Drake, 1992). Homeless, dually disordered persons generally fit poorly into existing mental health, substance abuse, and housing programs, and are unable to overcome the barriers between the three separate service systems (Drake, Osher et al., 1991).

Persons with dual disorders are strongly predisposed to homelessness, largely because their substance abuse and treatment noncompliance lead to disruptive behaviors, loss of social supports, and inability to maintain stable housing (Belcher, 1989; Benda and Datallo, 1988; Drake, Osher, and Wallach, 1989; Drake, Wallach, and Hoffman, 1989; Drake, Wallach et al., 1991; Lamb and Lamb, 1990). Once homeless, they have greater difficulties, require more services, and are more likely to remain homeless than other subgroups of homeless persons (Fischer, 1990). They are more likely to exhibit signs of psychological distress and deterioration, to trade sexual favors for food and money, to be estranged from their families, and to become incarcerated (Koegel and Burnam, 1987). They are also more likely to experience harsh conditions, such as living on the streets rather than in shelters (Fischer and Breakey, 1991). Standard mental health treatments are usually ineffective with this population, presumably because of insufficient intensity, unavailability of decent housing, and failure to address substance abuse effectively (Drake, Osher et al., 1991).

The Washington, D.C., Dual Diagnosis Project was initiated in 1990 to develop intensive, integrated services specifically tailored for homeless, dually diagnosed persons. The purposes of this paper are: (1) to describe this research demonstration project, and (2) to use this particular project to illustrate the use of a model-directed process evaluation in health services research.

PROJECT DESCRIPTION

The Washington, D.C., Dual Diagnosis Project is a research demonstration for homeless, dually diagnosed persons. The project takes place at

Community Connections, a private, nonprofit mental health agency located in southeast Washington, D.C. that provides comprehensive mental health services, including case management, psychotherapy, medications, rehabilitation, and housing, for approximately 300 adults with severe mental disorders. The central component of the Community Connections program is clinical case management (Harris and Bachrach, 1988). The program serves a predominantly minority population and specializes in the care of severely mentally disabled persons, especially homeless women. Homeless persons with severe psychiatric disabilities from throughout the District are eligible for referral. One of the co-directors of the organization, Maxine Harris, has been responsible for the design and maintenance of the two experimental models of intensive case management within Community Connections.

The research component of the project has been designed and directed by the New Hampshire-Dartmouth Psychiatric Research Center, a health services research group led by Robert Drake and Greg Teague, in collaboration with Howard University's Ernest Quimby, who has been responsible for the qualitative component. The project director for the on-site research team in Washington is Richard Bebout.

The project targets adults who are literally homeless (in shelters or on the streets) and dually diagnosed with severe mental illness and substance use disorder. Women have been purposely oversampled and comprise approximately 65% of the sample because women are usually underrepresented in studies of dual diagnosis and because the primary provider, Community Connections, has a long-standing commitment to serving severely mentally ill women. Consistent with the demographics of the local population, approximately 88% of the clients in the study are African-American.

The project includes two experimental models of intensive case management–Cognitive-Behavioral Treatment (CBT) and Social Network Treatment (SNT)–at Community Connections and a quasi-experimental comparison condition of standard treatment at D.C. community mental health centers (CMHCs). Clients referred to the project, who met study criteria and gave informed consent, were randomly assigned to the two experimental models, both of which are provided at Community Connections. The study examines process, clinical effectiveness, and cost-effectiveness over 18 months for the 168 homeless, dually diagnosed clients who were assigned to either CBT or SNT. Because local CMHCs were unable to accept new referrals, thereby precluding random assignment, a comparison group of 75 clients who were already receiving services in the local CMHCs and substance abuse systems is being followed to assess clinical outcomes over 18 months. The nonexperimental comparison group was matched for age, gender, race, dual diagnosis, and history of homelessness with the two experimental groups.

The two experimental interventions, CBT and SNT, share several features: Both prescribe clinical case management as the central catalyst to change and recovery. Both teams have small caseloads (one clinician per 15 clients) and provide outreach and frequent contacts to engage clients. They attempt to meet basic needs as a precondition for treatment. And in each model, the same treatment team addresses housing, substance abuse treatment, and mental health treatment concurrently, so that providers, rather than clients, assume the burden of integrating multiple systems of care (Kline, Harris, Bebout, and Drake, 1991).

The two experimental models overlap extensively with respect to the basic service delivery model and resources available. CBT and SNT differ, however, in the proposed mechanism of change: Cognitive-Behavioral Treatment directly addresses the knowledge, attitudes, beliefs, and habits that sustain substance abuse and attempts to substitute new cognitions and behaviors that will support abstinence. Treatment occurs largely in individual and group counseling sessions in the clinic. By contrast, Social Network Treatment focuses on social and other environmental cues and reinforcers, and assumes that substance abuse can be reduced in disorganized and psychotic clients by changing their environments and social networks. Treatment occurs largely in network meetings in the community.

The project will test several specific hypotheses (Drake, Bebout, and Roach, 1993). First, CBT and SNT will be superior to standard community services in several respects, particularly in reducing substance abuse and improving the stability of housing. Second, the two experimental conditions will differentially affect some specific outcomes, such as SNT improving social networks and CBT affecting knowledge and attitudes toward substance abuse. Third, the two experimental interventions will differentially impact on clients based on their characteristics. For example, SNT will be more successful with clients who have cognitive impairments, and CBT will be more effective with those who have a good learning capacity.

The Washington, D.C., Dual Diagnosis Project began recruiting clients and providing services in 1991. Recruitment was completed in July, 1992. To preserve statistical power, outcome data will not be examined until all subjects have completed 18 months. However, clinicians and researchers in this project have been using data from the process analysis extensively. The remainder of this report will be devoted to describing the process evaluation.

PROCESS EVALUATION

The terms implementation evaluation, program monitoring, and process evaluation are used interchangeably by different authors (Teague, Schwab, and Drake, 1990). All refer to attempts to measure the program itself, as opposed to its effects or outcomes. Brekke (1987) has described an approach similar to the one used here as model-guided process evaluation. Though often neglected, a process evaluation serves several critical functions, e.g., to define the treatment model, to assess the fidelity of the implementation, and to inform the outcome evaluation. Evaluating the process of service delivery entails a series of logical steps. These include specifying the model, implementing the model, monitoring the integrity of the model over time, assessing the extent of exposure to and absorption of the intervention, and using the process data to understand clients' intermediate steps as well as final outcomes. Several mechanisms are being used to evaluate the process in this study.

Specifying the Model

The central feature of model implementation for clinical and services research is a detailed treatment manual that guides the delivery of services. A treatment manual aids training, supervision, and monitoring of services by operationalizing basic theoretical concepts and by specifying interventions. Concrete guidelines and clinical examples allow the project to achieve consistency across practitioners and stability over time. Treatment manuals also allow for valid replications in other settings.

For this project, both CBT and SNT developed detailed treatment manuals during the early phases. The CBT manual, for example, specifies individual and group interventions for aiding clients in identifying and breaking the links between internal and external risk factors and substance abuse. Using case examples, it illustrates how a cognitive-behavioral therapist intervenes in a variety of typical situations. The SNT manual offers similarly concrete guidelines for assessing networks, establishing new social connections, and correcting difficulties in current networks.

Implementation

Master's level clinicians with experience treating persons who have long-term mental illness were recruited for both experimental conditions. Preference was given to clinicians who had worked with homeless persons. Clinicians with a preference for direct counseling and cognitive-behavioral interventions were selected for the CBT model, and those with interests in an ecological perspective and social networks were selected for the SNT model.

Initial training of case managers began with an intensive apprenticeship. Each new case manager worked closely with the team supervisor or a senior case manager. Case managers received three hours per week of individual supervision for the first three months. Since then, they have received individual and group supervision weekly from the team leaders, who are experts in the respective models. In addition, these team leaders are available daily to provide brief consultations and to help in conducting emergency, group, or network interventions. This level of contact aids the process analysis because supervisors are inevitably involved in the clinical effort as participant-observers, helping with an intervention but also observing supervisees. Finally, each team meets every six weeks with the program director and the on-site research project director for a half-day retreat to discuss their clinical work and observations working within the model.

Monitoring Clinician Behavior

Case manager activity logs, modeled on logs developed by the research team in New Hampshire (Teague et al., 1990), were modified specifically for the purposes of this project. These logs are used on a time-sampling basis, so that each case manager fills out an activity log during one complete week of each month. Our prior research has established that case managers are able to provide accurate information on daily activities for the previous week and that time-sampling allows for the stable construction of an individual case manager's and a team's activities (Teague, Drake, McKenna, and Schwab, 1991). These logs are purposely simplified to document activities, participants, and the location of activities that are model-specific and that differentiate between the two experimental models. For example, individual sessions for cognitive mapping regarding substance abuse should be much more common in the CBT model, while network meetings with housing companions should predominate in the SNT model. Service log data are immediately computerized and shared with team supervisors to help in the process of identifying model noncompliance or drift. For example, service log data reveal that CBT case managers spend less than 2% of their time with network members, whereas SNT case managers devote more than 40% of their time to activities that involve members of clients' networks.

Research assistants regularly review all clinical records to collect data regarding drug tests, case manager ratings, and service utilization. This process allows for a routine check on the details of planning, delivering, and documenting treatment. Any activities that indicate discrepancies from the model are identified for review by the research project director and the program director.

Measuring Service Utilization

We review utilization data gathered from several reporting mechanisms. A version of the Treatment Services Review (McLellan, Luborsky, O'Brien, and Woody, 1992), which was specifically adapted for this project by NIAAA, is included as part of the follow-up interviews every six months. The Treatment Services Review allows the client to report services received in the eight categories of need taken from the Addiction Severity Index (McLellan, Luborsky, O'Brien, and Woody, 1980). In the version used for this project, the client reports the number of days that services were received during the previous 60 days.

Both interventions prescribe group activities as a central defining feature. For the CBT intervention, these involve substance abuse treatment groups in the treatment center such as the Psychoeducation Group and the Problems of Living Group; the SNT model relies heavily on network meetings in the community such as Residential Nework Groups and Multiple Family Groups. In each case attendance logs are maintained as a measure of exposure to the model.

Quarterly Report Forms, developed by NIAAA and participating researchers to report service utilization across all study sites, indicate whether specific categories of services (5 broad categories and 39 subcategories) were provided to each client during each three-month interval. For the purposes of process evaluation, the data give a gross indication of whether services that are model-specific predominate in the expected 3:1 or greater ratio within each model and whether services that are not model-specific are equivalent across the two models. Any deviations from these findings would be explored with finer data and discussed with supervisors.

Stability of housing is a key outcome variable for this study, but the use of various housing resources is also a critical aspect of the process evaluation. Clients in both conditions have access to a broad continuum of housing services that range from individualized supported housing to highly structured, congregate living situations (Bebout and Harris, 1992). Movements through this system, as well as exits and returns to homelessness and institutional settings, are monitored carefully, and clinicians document on standardized forms the circumstances surrounding transitions.

Model Absorption

To assess whether or not clients who are exposed to a model absorb the elements that are presumed to be effective, intermediate changes (often termed proximal effects) that are specified by the logic of each model are tested. For example, in the CBT model, clients are expected to develop a close, working relationship with their case managers, to internalize information about drug abuse, and to learn specific cognitive strategies related to avoiding drug abuse. To evaluate these intermediate outcomes, interviews incorporate modified forms of the Working Alliance Inventory (Horvath and Greenberg, 1989), the Drinking Related I-E Scale (Donovan and O'Leary, 1978) and the Situational Confidence Questionnaire (Annis and Graham, 1988). In the SNT intervention, intermediate changes in the social network should be apparent. Specifically, substance-abusing network members should begin to disappear, while more network members who are not substance abusers should begin to appear. To evaluate this transitional process, clients are asked about their social networks in a structured manner based on the Social Support and Social Network Inventory (Lovell, Barrow, and Hammer, 1984).

Qualitative Approaches

In addition to quantitative approaches to understanding process, our ethnographic team has worked intensively with a subset of 25 clients to attempt to understand their perceptions, attitudes, and experiences regarding substance abuse and treatment in greater depth. These clients are followed weekly whether they are in treatment or not, in housing or not. Qualitative methods include participant-observation, semi-structured interviews with the clients and their network members, and focus groups.

Qualitative data can aid the interpretation of quantitative data and provide insights into areas that are not addressed specifically by the quantitative approaches. For example, the quantitative data in this study will assess how often a particular case manager and client meet and what activities they are engaged in, but not why the relationship succeeds or fails. Qualitative approaches are intended to enhance our understanding of the nature of the case manager-client relationships and how they develop within each model. How does the client experience these interventions? What perceived attitudes and behaviors of the case manager enhance or impede the development of a working alliance? How do sociocultural factors influence the client's experience, particularly when the case manager and client come from different racial backgrounds? How does the client view treatment, housing, social networks, and recovery?

USES OF PROCESS DATA

In this section we will illustrate some of the ways in which process data can be helpful prior to the stage of interpreting clinical outcomes.

Clarifying the Boundaries Between Interventions

Clinical demonstrations are plagued by tendencies for models to evolve and drift during the course of studies. Treatment manuals enable clinicians, supervisors, and evaluators to be specific and consistent about what constitutes the intervention and what represents drift or cross-over to another intervention. The clinical staff themselves need to be involved in developing these manuals to ensure that behaviors and interventions are explicit rather than abstract. Manuals that focus exclusively on mission, values, and principles do not permit empirical monitoring and replication in new sites.

In this project, specific clinical vignettes were discussed extensively to define the boundaries between the two experimental interventions. Discussing the same vignettes separately with each team allowed the program director to clarify the differences in approach, ensure that the interventions were consistent with the models, document these differences in the treatment manuals, and hold clinical supervisors and clinicians responsible for adhering to the respective models.

Improving Model Adherence

One case manager provided data on a variety of reporting forms that were discrepant from those of other team members and inconsistent with the treatment manual. Close supervision and observation determined that this case manager had strong biases about treatment that precluded adherence to the model. He was therefore transferred to another case management team outside of the project, and a new case manager was recruited.

A second case manager was identified through the logs as drifting toward the comparison model. In this instance, an SNT case manager was high in direct counseling and low in social network interventions. Feedback and clinical supervision corrected the behaviors, and the supervisor's observations confirmed model adherence. Longitudinal monitoring showed that this case manager's activities became similar to those of his team members and were significantly different from CBT case managers' activities on key dimensions such as providing network meetings outside of the clinic and accompanying clients to Alcoholics Anonymous meetings.

The research protocol specified that urine drug screens were to be obtained on a random basis at least every three months, but process data revealed that drug screens were not regularly obtained for over half of the clients in both conditions early in the course of the study. Further followup revealed that concern about the treatment alliance was a major factor contributing to noncompliance. Case managers' assistance improved when the drug-screening was reframed as a study requirement rather than a clinical judgment. The proportion of clients receiving random drug screens improved substantially to more than 80% of active treatment cases.

Understanding the Clinical Relationship and Attrition

Qualitative data and ratings of the case manager-client relationship through structured questionnaires enabled the research team to understand the extent of clients' ambivalence toward the control and authority exercised by case managers. Using either assessment alone would have been insufficient to understand some aspects of attrition.

Process data showed that clients have a tendency to rate the relationship with their case manager highly from the beginning of the relationship, while case managers' ratings of the same relationships decline slightly over the first several months and correspond poorly with the clients' ratings over time. Ethnographic studies of case management in this project and others have helped to explain this finding by documenting the extent to which clients are ambivalent about case managers' perceived power, authority, and control of resources. Many clients feel compelled to distort their responses, even on research interviews, in order to maximize their chances of obtaining needed resources. Over time case managers become more aware of this process and more realistic about the extent of ambivalence and the quality of collaboration. Some clients entered the project in order to obtain access to resources–e.g., help with entitlements, housing, and medical care–but did not intend to modify their destructive behaviors toward others and themselves. They often became early dropouts.

Studying Housing Models

The circumstances surrounding transitions in living situations and stable housing arrangements have allowed the research team to understand several aspects of housing arrangements for homeless, dually diagnosed clients. Clients frequently prefer single-unit apartments in the community rather than structured or congregate living situations, but single apartments rarely provide social network support for abstinence and often provide peer-pressure and opportunities for continuance or renewal of substance abuse. Despite numerous placements in these kinds of arrangements and extensive outreach by Community Connections staff, few clients have been able to maintain these types of supported housing arrangements. Instead, they typically encounter difficulties related to alcohol, drugs, or disruptive behaviors and return to homeless shelters or institutional situations after brief stays. In contrast, clients who agree to structured living arrangements of various types, usually congregate living situations, are more likely to develop networks of friends who are not addicted to drugs, to attain stability themselves, and to maintain community tenure.

CONCLUSION

A model-guided process evaluation critically informs health services research demonstrations. It enables the researchers to interpret outcomes, since neither positive nor negative results can be understood in the absence of a process evaluation. A carefully designed analysis of process also facilitates implementation and maintenance of the model, and materials used in and deriving from this analysis ensure replicability. We have used our Washington, D.C., Dual Diagnosis Project to illustrate a specific application of these methods. Other studies would of course require different measures, but the basic approach to process evaluation is similar.

REFERENCES

Annis, H.M., & Graham, J.M. (1988). *Situational Confidence Questionnaire (SCQ-39): User's guide.* Toronto: Addiction Research Foundation.

Bebout, R.R., & Harris, M. (1992). In search of pumpkin shells: Residential programming for the homeless mentally ill. In H.R. Lamb, L.L. Bachrach, & F.I. Kass (Eds.), *Treating the homeless mentally ill* (pp. 159-181). Washington, D.C.: American Psychiatric Press.

Belcher, J.R. (1989). On becoming homeless: A study of chronically mentally ill persons. *Journal of Community Psychology, 17,* 173-185.

Benda, B.B., & Datallo, P. (1988). Homelessness: Consequence of a crisis or a long-term process? *Hospital and Community Psychiatry, 39,* 884-886.

Brekke, J.S. (1987). The model-guided method of monitoring program implementation. *Evaluation Review, 11,* 281-300.

Donovan, D.M., & O'Leary, M.R. (1978). The drinking-related locus of control scale: Reliability, factor structure, and validity. *Journal of Studies on Alcohol, 39,* 759-780.

Drake, R.E., Bebout, R.R., & Roach, J.P. (1993). A research evaluation of social network case management for homeless persons with dual disorders. In M. Harris & H. Bergman (Eds.), *Case management: Theory and practice.* New York: Harwood Press, 83-98.

Drake, R.E., Osher, F.C., & Wallach, F.C. (1989). Alcohol use and abuse in schizophrenia: A prospective community study. *Journal of Nervous and Mental Disease, 177,* 408-414.

Drake, R.E., Osher, F.C., & Wallach, F.C. (1991). Homelessness and dual diagnosis. *American Psychologist, 46,* 1149-1158.

Drake, R.E., & Wallach, M.A. (1992). Mental patients' attraction to the hospital: Correlates of living preference. *Community Mental Health Journal, 28,* 5-12.

Drake, R.E., Wallach, M.A., & Hoffman, J.S. (1989). Housing instability and homelessness among aftercare patients of an urban state hospital. *Hospital and Community Psychiatry, 40,* 46-51.

Drake, R.E., Wallach, M.A., Teague, G.B., Freeman, D.H., Paskus, T.S., & Clark, T.A. (1991). Housing instability and homelessness among rural schizophrenic patients. *American Journal of Psychiatry, 148,* 330-336.

Fischer, P.J. (1990). *Alcohol and drug abuse and mental health problems among homeless persons: A review of the literature, 1980-1990.* Rockville, MD: National Institutes on Alcohol Abuse and Alcoholism.

Fischer, P.J., & Breakey, W.R. (1991, May). *Correlates of homelessness in a Baltimore dual diagnosed population.* Paper presented at the annual meeting of the American Psychiatric Association, New Orleans, LA.

Harris, M., & Bachrach, L.L. (Eds.) (1988). *New directions in clinical case management.* San Francisco: Jossey-Bass.

Horvath, A.O., & Greenberg, L.S. (1989). Development and validation of the Working Alliance Inventory. *Journal of Counseling Psychology, 36,* 223-233.

Kline, J., Harris, M., Bebout, R.R., & Drake, R.E. (1991). Contrasting integrated and linkage models of treatment for homeless, dually diagnosed adults. In K. Minkoff & R.E. Drake (Eds.), *Dual diagnosis of major mental illness and substance disorder* (pp. 95-106). San Francisco: Jossey-Bass.

Koegel, P., & Burnam, M.A. (1987). *The epidemiology of alcohol abuse and dependence among the homeless: Findings from the inner city of Los Angeles.* Rockville, MD: National Institute on Alcohol Abuse and Alcoholism.

Lamb, H.R., & Lamb, D.M. (1990). Factors contributing to homelessness among the chronically and severely mentally ill. *Hospital and Community Psychiatry, 41,* 301-305.

Lovell, A.M., Barrow, S., & Hammer, M. (1984). *Social Support and Social Network Interview.* New York: New York State Psychiatric Institute.

McLellan, A.T., Alterman, A.I., Cacciola, J., Metzger, D., & O'Brien, C.P. (1992). A new measure of substance abuse treatment: Initial studies of the Treatment Services Review. *Journal of Nervous and Mental Disease, 180,* 101-110.

McLellan, A.T., Luborsky, L., O'Brien, C.P., & Woody, G.E. (1980). An improved evaluation instrument for substance abuse patients: The Addiction Severity Index. *Journal of Nervous and Mental Disease, 168,* 826-833.

Minkoff, K., & Drake, R.E. (1992). Homelessness and dual diagnosis. In H.R. Lamb, L.L. Bachrach, & F.I. Kass (Eds.), *Treating the homeless mentally ill* (pp. 221-247). Washington, D.C.: American Psychiatric Press.

Teague, G.B., Drake, R.E., McKenna, P. & Schwab, B. (1991, June). *Implementation evaluation related to continuous treatment teams for dually diagnosed persons in New Hampshire.* Paper presented at the NIMH Community Support Program Conference, Rockville, MD.

Teague, G.B., Schwab, B., & Drake, R.E. (1990). *Evaluating services for young adults with severe mental illness and substance use disorders.* Arlington, VA: National Association of State Mental Health Program Directors.

OUTREACH: SEATTLE

Systems Alliance and Support (SAS): A Program of Intensive Case Management for Chronic Public Inebriates: Seattle

Gary B. Cox, PhD
Lucia Meijer
Donna I. Carr, MS, QCDC
Steven A. Freng, MSW

Gary B. Cox is a member of the faculty of the Department of Psychiatry and Behavioral Sciences RP-10, University of Washington, Seattle, WA 98195. Lucia Meijer is Program Administrator, Donna I. Carr is Program Supervisor, and Steven A. Freng is Division Manager, all with the King County Division of Alcohol and Substance Abuse Services.

Support for this project was provided by cooperative agreement U01 AA08798, from the National Institute on Alcohol Abuse and Alcoholism.

[Haworth co-indexing entry note]: "Systems Alliance and Support (SAS): A Program of Intensive Case Management for Chronic Public Inebriates: Seattle." Cox, Gary B. et al. Co-published simultaneously in the *Alcoholism Treatment Quarterly* (The Haworth Press, Inc.) Vol. 10, No. 3/4, 1993, pp. 125-138; and: *Treatment of the Chemically Dependent Homeless: Theory and Implementation in Fourteen American Projects* (ed: Kendon J. Conrad, Cheryl I. Hultman, and John S. Lyons) The Haworth Press, Inc., 1993, pp. 125-138. Multiple copies of this article/chapter may be purchased from The Haworth Document Delivery Center [1-800-3-HAWORTH: 9:00 a.m. - 5:00 p.m. (EST)].

SUMMARY. Systems Alliance and Support (SAS) is a long-term, intensive case management intervention suitable for severely disabled chronic alcoholics. These clients have long histories of alcohol abuse and of unsuccessful treatment for alcoholism, and for our subjects, long histories of homelessness, with a paucity of personal resources or reserves to assist in recovery. Given these characteristics, we expect these clients to move only very slowly and in small increments toward recovery, and to be prone to relapse. The goals of our intervention are to help stabilize the clients' lives by assisting in basic support areas such as financial aid and housing, and subsequently to help them reduce or cease alcohol consumption.

BACKGROUND

King County, Washington, which includes the City of Seattle, contains about forty percent of the population of the State. Publicly funded drug and alcohol services for the county and the various metropolitan areas within it, are provided by the King County Division of Alcohol and Substance Abuse Services (DASAS). The service system is an exemplar of the "continuity of care" service model, with a full range of standard detoxification, residential, outpatient, and aftercare service components.

The King County Detoxification Center (KCDC) is an integral part of this system. It is the only medical model detoxification facility in western Washington, and as such has traditionally served not only the clients of King County, but on demand those of surrounding jurisdictions. For many years this worked well, in that the facility had sufficient capacity to meet all these service needs. In recent years, however, demand for services has grown to the point that not all persons needing admittance could be accepted. In keeping with the pattern typical for such facilities (Finn, 1985), the DASAS noted that a small number of clients accounted for a large number of KCDC admissions, and administrators began to consider ways to increase the number of clients who could be served by reducing the number of admissions for these high frequency users.

In 1987, when NIAAA released its first round of Demonstration Projects for Homeless Substance Abusing Persons, King County proposed to provide intensive case management to a sample of homeless high frequency detoxification users. The rationale for this choice of intervention was that these clients had already experienced virtually every type of standard approach to treatment available, often multiple times, with no positive results, so that if there was to be any hope for improvement, a new approach was needed. This proposal was not funded, but the County was able to find enough money for a small pilot version of the intervention. This study showed significant changes in the targeted outcomes, increased financial and residential stability, and reduced admissions to the Detoxification facility (Freng, Carr & Cox, 1992). Unfortunately these results were based on a relatively weak, pre-post design, with no other control condition. A related outcome, however, was that by the time the second round research demonstration proposals were solicited by NIAAA, the DASAS had about two years of experience with case management for this population. When NIAAA announced a second round of projects to address the needs of homeless, substance abusing persons, staff from DASAS initiated a collaboration with faculty from the University of Washington which led to a proposal that was funded.

OBJECTIVES

The target population for this intervention is "chronic public inebriates," defined in this case as persons who are high frequency users of the King County Detoxification Center ("Detox"). This group was selected because of its high level of consumption of resources (Wells, 1985) and lack of responsiveness to standard treatments, and the consequent fact that a large increase in treatment resources could be made available if these clients reduced their utilization (Kivlahan et al., 1985). Administratively, then, a major outcome of interest would be reduced Detox admissions for members of the case managed group.

We assumed that alcohol would be the primary drug of abuse for most, but not necessarily all, of these persons, that many of them would have long histories of substance abuse and of treatment for their abuse, that they would be predominantly homeless or at risk for homelessness (for purposes of the grant, only these Ss could be served), and that they would be severely disabled with few personal resources available to aid in their recovery or in the maintenance of any gains made toward recovery.

These assumptions have several implications. First, if the clients are immersed in a substance or alcohol abuse oriented street subculture, then change will be extremely difficult to accomplish so long as they remain in that setting. Second, given their (often) long histories of abuse, not uncommonly with a lack of history of successful adjustment in society, abstinence is probably not a goal they are likely to attain, much less maintain, in a short period of time. Third, their level of habituation and disability suggests that a long period of support will be required if abstinence, or even substantial reductions in drinking, are to be achieved and maintained (Institute of Medicine, 1990).

The overall objectives of the intervention, then, are twofold. The first and most immediately attainable goal is to reduce the harmful effects associated with chronic substance use, including homelessness, illness, personal victimization, and criminal activity. This requires introducing an element of stability and certainty into an otherwise chaotic lifestyle by providing the client with assistance in basic life-support areas such as financial aid, housing, health care, household management and so forth. The second and more elusive goal is to help the clients reduce, and preferably cease, their consumption of alcohol and other drugs.

THE INTERVENTION:
SYSTEMS ALLIANCE AND SUPPORT (SAS)

Both these goals are approached in the context of intense, long-term support, oriented toward strengthening the personal and social skills of the clients. In the intermediate time frame, a goal is to reduce clients' need for Detox and other acute care services, and in the longer run, to substantially reduce or eliminate harmful substance use.

Most treatment approaches take the position that the life problems experienced by the chronic alcoholic are the direct or indirect result of the addiction. This philosophy mandates immediate and ongoing focus on drinking behaviors based on the belief that if you can't stop the drinking, nothing else can get better. Unfortunately, in the case of the chronically disabled alcoholic, many of the problems associated with drinking are in turn barriers to treatment. Poor health, lack of housing, and a chaotic, transient lifestyle can make it extremely difficult to access many services, and in turn reduce the likelihood of the client being interested in or responsive to treatment. Moreover, not all the alcoholic's life problems are a by-product of his/her chronic drinking. In many cases they are co-factors in a larger picture of life-long pervasive physical, psychological, and social dysfunction.

Our intervention differs from standard treatment in several ways. First it is all individual, no groups are involved. Group activities require a level of commitment, skills, trust, and stability not typically found in this population. Second, it is not, at least initially and not centrally, focussed on drinking. Rather the case managers help the clients deal with a wide range of problems in their life situations. Most clients are quickly alienated by an approach that prioritizes their drinking behaviors over their more immediately felt problems. Third, the ongoing provision of case management is never made contingent on the client stopping or reducing drinking. Rather the focus is on sustaining a positive connection with the client that carries the potential, but not the requirement, for eventual movement towards a drug-free lifestyle. Fourth, the intervention is long-term. We expect to retain Ss in case management for the duration of the research project. At the end of funding, case managed clients will have received between 20 and 30 months of these services.

Program values stress the importance of assuring client survival needs using the least intrusive measures possible. The client's continued involvement in the program is of primary importance, regardless of his/her progress or lack thereof. Helping the client achieve increased levels of self-management is more important than the case manager taking action to assure stability in every aspect of the client's life. Clients are encouraged to learn self-management skills even at the risk of occasional failure. There are no punishments attached to failure, but clients are expected to deal with the consequences of their actions.

Concretely, the case managers engage in the activities that are traditional for case management: they assess and prioritize the client's needs, assess the client's strengths and resources, locate needed resources, assist the client in overcoming barriers to accessing these resources, attempt to motivate the client, provide advocacy for the client with other services, coordinate multiple services, and monitor the services and client to ensure follow-up and compliance. All of these activities are guided by two principles. The first is that clients should be given every opportunity to meet their own needs. We attempt to encourage client participation and autonomy by such mechanisms as encouraging the client to set his/her own service plan objectives and be involved in treatment planning, and encouraging the client to perform necessary tasks himself/herself. Only if the client is unable to accomplish a task should the case manager help directly with it.

The second principle is a focus on incremental rather than radical change. We begin with a minimal level of intervention, and observe the client's ability to manage at that level of interpersonal relations, personal hygiene, independent living, or whatever. We provide extensive encouragement for any behavior approximating improved functioning, and move on to a higher level only as the client appears to be ready to handle the new responsibilities.

Although there are variations in how case management is conceived (Bachrach, 1992; Grahm & Birchmore-Timney, 1989), the model we are describing is well within standard descriptions (Intaglia, 1982; O'Connor, 1988). Nor are we the first to propose it in the treatment of alcoholism (Sternbach, 1982; Willenbring, 1990) or substance abuse (McCarty et al., 1991; Birchmore-Timney & Grahm, 1989). Still, case management represents a relatively new idea with no established credentials in these fields. The Institute of Medicine's (1990) comprehensive report on alcoholism, for example, does not mention case management in its chapter reviewing treatment.

IMPLEMENTATION

Starting the Program

Case Management is a relatively easy program to initiate. The major start-up task is to hire staff. Since there is no in-house or group treatment program, and since staff spend much time in the streets, physical space needs are minimal considering the number of staff and clients involved. Similarly, logistic, organizational, and system linkage demands are minimal: there are no medical, food, or other services for which supplies must be organized and coordinated, no necessity for tight staff, client or space schedules, and no need for coordinating committees with wide community and service program representation convened in order to avoid turf wars. The major requirement, and it is crucial, is administrative support.

Relationships with Other Programs

Part of the start-up period does involve establishing linkages, both formal and informal, with existing service providers. However, these do not have to be developed before the program can begin to function, and as the program operates, at least the informal ties will automatically strengthen to the extent that the case managers are effective. Other programs have generally reacted favorably to SAS. Partly this is due to the feeling that "it's about time someone started working with those people," and partly to more general common interests among service providers. It also helps if the case management program develops a reputation for effectiveness. One structured approach to establishing linkages has been for SAS and another service program to exchange program description presentations at staff meetings. In some cases where a particular service is important but difficult to master (e.g., SSI applications), one or two case managers will make an effort to become experts in that area for the group.

Staffing and Supervision

Case managers are hired for their ability to work with a highly impaired population, under a minimum of rules and regulations. Case managers must be familiar with the population, often through previous experience in shelter, Detox, emergency rooms or other facilities that typically work with these clients. They must be knowledgeable about chemical dependency, but be willing to accept the premise of an alternative service that does not necessarily require a commitment to abstinence. Case managers must be able to function independently in a variety of street and agency settings, including shelters, parks, and hotels. This means that they must be trained in personal safety skills and teamwork (they go in pairs in settings where there is any potential for personal hazard). Case managers must also be able to communicate effectively with service providers, law enforcement, and community business interests to advocate for clients and secure services. This dual role is particularly demanding since many people who are skilled with clients at the street level do not relate well in professional settings and vice versa.

Typically new case managers are assigned to a veteran case manager and quickly immersed in the daily routine. Most case managers learn by observing and then doing. Typically two to three months is required before case managers can be considered ready to function independently. There are few written protocols, and case managers must be able to adapt quickly to changing client situations and resources based on what they know about program philosophy and basic operating principles. Hiring has not presented any major obstacles, and new case managers appear to adjust well to the tasks.

This approach, although accepted and supported, can also create stress for case managers, who sometimes would like to have more structure, rules and procedures. In the absence of strict protocols and structure it is necessary for case managers to communicate with each other frequently and in great detail to ensure continuity of care and coordination of activities. This level of interaction is accomplished by a daily staff meeting. However, some case managers find this amount of interchange uncomfortable, time consuming and cumbersome. Also, because case management activities are driven by client needs rather than a structured program protocol, case managers often feel a lack of predictability in their work life. Intensely stressful activities involving critical interventions may alternate with periods of relative calm.

These stresses have been handled, at least in part, through the recent development of a self-managing team model in which staff take responsibility for most of the day-to-day operating decisions. This allows staff to experience a sense of control over their working lives and to communicate with each other in a manner that they find most useful.

Staff activities include (a) client assessment, (b) advocacy and coordination of services, (c) "home" visits (could be in a park, on a street corner, in a hotel, etc.), (d) resource development (negotiating with landlords, service providers, shelters, welfare, etc., for client services), (e) financial management (disbursement and monitoring of funds, food coupons, and other resources), (f) training clients in life-skills (e.g., assisting clients with shopping, laundry, housekeeping, obtaining showers, haircuts, clothing, etc.), (g) record keeping, and (h) client tracking (locating missing clients).

Some clients are seen several times a week while others are seen only a few times a month. Case managers maintain a "hot list" of clients who have not made recent contact, and actively try to locate them. While some staff activities take place regularly (e.g., staff meetings, office coverage, site visits, etc.), many activities are scheduled on an as-needed basis.

Caseloads are currently 15 clients per case manager. Within any case load there may be a wide range of need, with some clients receiving almost daily attention, and others requiring only occasional contacts. Most clients are assigned haphazardly to case managers. Case managers, however, often develop particular strengths, and clients who are seen to have special needs will be assigned to a case manager with matching strengths. Occasionally a client will be reassigned, either because unusual new needs are detected, or because a client forms an inappropriate attachment to the case manager.

As a rule clients respond to SAS services positively with varying degrees of caution and trust. Only a few clients have become behavior problems. Only when all possible approaches to work with the client have failed is termination from the project considered. This has happened with only three clients to date (of 150), and each case involved actual or threatened physical violence, extreme verbal abuse, and/or an extreme degree of uncooperativeness.

Financial Management

A major component of the program is the establishment of "protective payee" status whenever possible for the clients' disability payments. Certain programs, notably SSI, require that if a person's qualifying disability is due to drug or alcohol abuse, the payments must be made to a third party who will assist the payee in managing the funds. This allows clients to continue to function in the community even when they are too incapacitated by their alcoholism to continue to function independently. SAS has an accountant whose responsibility it is to actually handle the monthly checks and disbursement of funds for clients, approximately half the total caseload, for whom SAS has this relationship. The case managers, then, consult with the client to set a budget and control spending, and the case managers make requests to the accountant to obtain the funds. This is an extremely important mechanism for helping clients learn self-management skills. As long as other services are provided unconditionally, the potential for coercive use of protective payee status is limited. However, it is necessary to constantly reinforce program values concerning client autonomy and the use of least intrusive measures possible, in order to assure the principles are not violated.

RESEARCH DESIGN

Our research design called for recruiting 60 women (the FEM group), 120 Native American males (the NAM group), and 120 other, ethnically mixed, males (the OM group), for a total of 300 subjects. The target population was to be homeless chronic public inebriates, defined as those persons who used the Detox facility with high frequency. However, since we were deliberately oversampling women and Native American males, the criteria for frequency of Detox use varied across the three groups: for women and Native American males, 4 Detox admissions in the prior 12 months were required, for the other male group, 10 admissions in the prior 12 months. A list of eligible persons was maintained, and when a candidate was readmitted to Detox, s/he was invited to join the study. If s/he agreed, an interview was administered, the *S* was randomly assigned to case management or to treatment as usual, and, if assigned to case management, was introduced to the case management team. All *S*s were to be reinterviewed at six month intervals for the duration of the project, and those assigned to case management were to continue to receive that service for the duration of the project. Subjects were recruited in the period from March to December, 1991.

In practice we found that not enough Native American males were available to fill out that sample (in substantial measure because 30 of them were ineligible due to participation in the pilot study), so the OM group was expanded to complete the total sample. In addition, in order to fill out the final subjects, the required admission criteria were relaxed slightly for a few *S*s in each group. The final subgroup sample sizes were FEM = 57 (including 32 white and 20 Native American subjects), NAM = 78, and OM = 163 (100 white, 44 black and 19 Hispanic), for a total sample of 298. Random assignment to case management or treatment as usual was independent within subgroups.

CLIENT CHARACTERISTICS

Table 1 lists means (and standard deviations) and percentages for some basic descriptive characteristics. The subjects are notable for the severity

Table 1: Descriptive Characteristics of the Three Sample Subgroups			
	FEMALES (N=57)	NATIVE AMERICAN MALES (N=77)	OTHER MALES (N=164)
Mean Age	39.6(9.5)[1]	44.9(12.0)	43.1(10.0)
% Completed High School	61	62	70
% Married	12	5	5
% Never Married	35	39	37
Mean Number Detox Admissions in Prior 12 mos	5.5	19.6	26.4
Mean Number Years Use of Alcohol to Intoxication	17.8(9.1)	23.8(11.5)	23.9(11.1)
Mean Number Days in Prior 30 Used Alcohol to Intoxication	18.0(12.4)	22.4(9.6)	23.6(8.5)
Mean Age First Homeless	27.6(10.5)	29.4(12.0)	29.4(12.3)
Mean Longest Single Episode of Homelessness (in months)	27.0(58)	59.1(80)	45.0(68)
Mean total time homeless (in months)	37.4(61)	96.6(100)	73.6(84)

[1]Standard Deviations in parentheses.

of their substance abuse problems and long histories of homelessness. Most subjects (97% of males and 70% of females) reported that alcohol was their most problematic substance. Women were more likely than males to report heroin (16% v 2%) or cocaine (7% v < 1%) as their most serious problem. Most subjects (75% of males, 64% of females) did not report a second problem substance, but among males who did, heroin (7%), cocaine (5%), amphetamines (4%) and cannabis (3%) were most common, in contrast to women, for whom cocaine (14%) and alcohol (9%) were most likely.

Subjects' family backgrounds also included substantial alcohol abuse. Among all males, 68% reported parents, 61% siblings, and 69% other relatives (grandparents, aunts or uncles) with alcohol problems. For women, the analogous figures were 70%, 61%, and 67%. Fifty-eight percent of the women and 28% of the men reported being physically abused, and 28% of the women and 3% of the men sexually abused.

All subjects met criteria for homelessness or risk for homelessness, and only a handful of potential subjects who met the other admission criterion were excluded because they were not homeless. Further, these subjects reported extensive histories of homelessness.

IMPLICATIONS FOR PRACTICE, RESEARCH AND POLICY

Preliminary results from our six-month follow-up data (with not all *Ss* interviewed) suggest that, relative to the control group, SAS clients have significantly increased their income, reduced the number of nights spent on the streets and in shelters, increased the number of nights spent in their own housing, and have fewer, but not statistically significantly fewer, Detox admissions. Other indices of consumption also show non-significant differences. While stronger results on consumption would have been welcome, this pattern is consistent with our expectations for the intervention: We expect that changes in life situation will have to precede reduction in drinking for most clients. We are therefore pleased to note the presence of the changes we would expect in the short term, and hope to see greater changes in drinking related measures later. Until these results become available, we can speculate on the implications of the program on the assumption that the expected pattern continues to hold.

Clinical Implications

If the pattern holds, then we would conclude that intensive case management has promise as an intervention for severely disabled chronic alcoholics. On the one hand this perhaps should not be surprising. Fifteen years ago a literature began to appear in mental health showing that community treatment was as efficacious for the chronically mentally ill as institutional placement, and that in fact many of these clients could respond quite well to intensive community programs (Bond et al., 1988; Stein & Test, 1980). Previously it had been notoriously difficult to get most community mental health centers to address the needs of this population, because of the stereotype that the clients were difficult or impossible to treat. It remained for creative and aggressive community programs to demonstrate otherwise. Clearly it requires less creativity to at least attempt a similar treatment philosophy with a similarly disabled alcoholic population, but we hope to find a similar level of response.

Research Implications

The fuller nature and extent of these effects remain under study. A complete understanding of the effects requires that research questions of several types be addressed, including, for example, the following.

1. Cost-effectiveness trade-offs. The caseloads in the present study are 15 per manager. This is a level of intensity which probably cannot be provided in the typical treatment system. While this is reasonable in a demonstration situation, to test whether the effect can be demonstrated, to be practical caseloads will probably have to be more on the order of 25 per staff person, the typical levels of intensity for many publicly funded (as opposed to research or research demonstration projects) mental health case management programs. It would be surprising if the results from a program with a moderate average caseload, such as 25, would be as favorable as those for a more intensive program, such as our 15. Assuming they were not, one approach to evaluating trade-offs between two programs, one of which is both more expensive and more effective, is to perform cost-effectiveness analyses, to determine the number of units of improvement per program dollar in the two alternatives.

2. Differential outcomes. The question will arise as to whether differences in outcomes are due to different styles, skills, types of training or experience, or whatever, of case managers, or of differences in client characteristics or motivation, or of interactions between the two. Such speculation is inevitable in view of the extent of interest and research effort being expended on "matching" currently in the alcohol and drug treatment literature. Certainly some clients will get better and others won't, so it is as useful to investigate matching in case management as anywhere. Done properly this would require a theory about which staff and client characteristics are salient, sets of staff and clients who would represent the range of required characteristics, and random assignment of clients to case managers. It is also possible that the important features are more in the program (e.g., the use of protective payee procedures) than staff or clients.

3. Longer term outcomes. We expect that our clients will take longer to respond than is usual in alcohol treatment programs, and that their response, at least in the early stages, may be less than complete. We do not know whether to expect that all the clients who are going to respond will begin to do so within, say, the first year, or whether some might begin to respond only after a much longer period of intervention. Neither do we know whether, among those who do respond, any gains made can be expected to be self maintained, or whether we should expect to have to provide maintenance support for a prolonged time.

4. Portability or adaptability of SAS. To what extent can the SAS model of case management be used elsewhere–e.g., to what extent is any case management program dependent on the service system context? Since the model we are suggesting is a variation of standard case management practice, we think the prospects for portability should be excellent, provided the treatment goals and approach we describe are philosophically acceptable. But again, if there are variations in how well case management works across multiple sites, research into the "active ingredients" in the intervention would be possible and interesting.

5. *Variations in model.* Some have been discussed above, e.g., variations in caseload, or differences in case managers or clientele. Other variations might be desirable enhancements or extensions to the model and/or to the treatment system. Possibilities include incorporating a residential program, GED training, job training, job placement, and mental health services. All of these are reasonable considerations, given the characteristics of the sample as described above. In fact, it could be argued that unless some of these are added, especially job training and mental health services, it is not reasonable to expect long term successful outcomes for many clients in this group.

Policy Implications

Assuming some level of positive results for our study, the implications for policy for other service systems would depend, among other things, on (a) the cost-effectiveness of the intervention, that is, on whether there are sufficient reductions in costs of Detox, emergency room services, jail episodes, and other services, to partially or substantially off-set the case management costs and the increases in other service costs that the case management facilitates, (b) the suitability of the new setting for the addition of case management, which is really appropriate only if enough other service resources are available for there to be something for the case managers to coordinate, and (c) most basically, whether community values in a new setting will support this philosophical approach to intervention with this population.

Prospects for Continuation

The King County Alcohol and Substance Abuse Administrative Board, which is the policy setting body for DASAS, in its draft for the 1993-95 biennial plan for services, has identified case management and support for the chronic public inebriate as among its very highest priority items. Thus the likelihood of some form of case management for our study population is extremely high. The exact form of the transition between the current and future funding is not clear, and it is likely that the caseloads will be higher. The content of the program, however, will almost certainly be as nearly like the current SAS as other constraints will permit.

REFERENCES

Bachrach, L. L. (1992). Case management revisited. *Hospital and Community Psychiatry, 43*, 209-210.

Birchmore-Timney, C. & Grahm, K. (1989). A survey of case management practices in addictions programs. *Alcoholism Treatment Quarterly, 6*, 103-127.

Bond, G. R., Miller, L. D., Krumweid, M. H. A., & Ward, R. S. (1988). Assertive case management in three CMHCs: A controlled study. *Hospital and Community Psychiatry, 39*, 411-418.

Finn, P. (1985). Decriminalization of public drunkenness: Response of the health care system. *Journal of Studies on Alcohol, 46*, 7-23.

Freng, S. A., Carr, D. I., & Cox, G. B. (1992). Intensive case management for chronic public inebriates: A pilot study. Unpublished manuscript.

Grahm, K., & Birchmore-Timney, C. (1989). The problem of replicability in program evaluation: The component solution using the example of case management. *Evaluation and Program Planning, 12*, 179-187.

Intagliata, J. (1982). Improving the quality of care for the chronically mentally disabled: The role of case management. *Schizophrenia Bulletin, 8*, 655-674.

Institute on Medicine. (1990). *Broadening the base of treatment for alcohol problems*. Washington, DC: National Academy Press.

Kivlahan, D. R., Walker, R. D., Donovan, D. M., & Mischke, H. D. (1985). Detoxification recidivism among urban American Indian alcoholics. *American Journal of Psychiatry, 142*, 1467-1470.

McCarty, D., Argeriou, M., Hoffman, M., Mulvey, K., & Hennen, J. (1991, November). *The effects of case management and treatment setting on the homeless substance abuser: A demonstration project.* Paper presented at the meeting of the American Public Health Association, Atlanta, GA.

O'Connor, G. G. (1988). Case management: System and practice. *Social Casework: The Journal of Contemporary Social Work, 69*, 97-106.

Stein, L. I., & Test, M. A. (1980). Alternative to mental hospital treatment: I. Conceptual model, treatment program, and clinical evaluation. *Archives of General Psychiatry, 37*, 392-397.

Sternbach, T. G. (1982). The recidivist alcoholic management program (RAMP): A high intensity case management approach to treating chronic recidivist alcoholics. In P. Golding (Ed.), *Alcoholism: A modern perspective.* Ridgewood, NJ: George A. Bogden & Son.

Wells, J. E. (1985). Recurrent alcoholism: Readmissions for treatment for alcoholism. *New Zealand Medical Journal, 98*, 500-503.

Willenbring, M. L., Whelan, J. A., Dahlquist, J. S., & O'Neal, M. E. (1990). Community treatment of the chronic public inebriate I: Implementation. *Alcoholism Treatment Quarterly, 7*, 79-97.

RESIDENTIAL CARE: ALBUQUERQUE, EVANSTON / VA, LOS ANGELES

Albuquerque's Community-Based Housing and Support Services Demonstration Program for Homeless Alcohol Abusers

Sandra C. Lapham, MD, MPH
Marge Hall, MA
Marsha McMurray-Avila, MA
Harry Beaman, MA

Sandra C. Lapham, Marge Hall, Marsha McMurray-Avila, and Harry Beaman are affiliated with the Lovelace Institute for Health & Population Research, Health Care for the Homeless, and St. Martin's Hospitality Center, Albuquerque, NM.

Address correspondence to: Sandra Lapham, Director, Substance Abuse Research Programs, Lovelace Institute for Health & Population Research, 1650 University S.E., Suite 302, Albuquerque, NM, 87102.

This research demonstration program is supported by grant AA08818, from the National Institutes on Alcohol Abuse and Alcoholism.

[Haworth co-indexing entry note]: "Albuquerque's Community-Based Housing and Support Services Demonstration Program for Homeless Alcohol Abusers." Lapham, Sandra C. et al. Co-published simultaneously in the *Alcoholism Treatment Quarterly* (The Haworth Press, Inc.) Vol. 10, No. 3/4, 1993, pp. 139-154; and: *Treatment of the Chemically Dependent Homeless: Theory and Implementation in Fourteen American Projects* (ed: Kendon J. Conrad, Cheryl I. Hultman, and John S. Lyons) The Haworth Press, Inc., 1993, pp. 139-154. Multiple copies of this article/chapter may be purchased from The Haworth Document Delivery Center [1-800-3-HAWORTH: 9:00 a.m. - 5:00 p.m. (EST)].

139

SUMMARY. Albuquerque's community-based housing and support services demonstration program is a prospective, randomized comparison of the efficacy of three intervention strategies for treating homeless persons with alcohol-related problems. The present paper defines the target population, describes the theoretical model underlying the intervention design, and provides descriptions of the interventions, which include the social model detoxification program established for the project and the extended intervention programs undergoing evaluation. The paper then identifies some of the unanticipated developments encountered in the early phases of the program and programmatic responses to these challenges. Lessons learned during this process are described, in hopes that they might prove useful to others striving to develop similar programs.

SETTING

New Mexico, although the fifth largest state geographically, has only 1.5 million residents (U.S. Census, 1990). This state embodies a rich cultural diversity and heritage. National census figures (1990) reveal that New Mexico has the highest percentage of residents of Hispanic origin (40%) and the second highest percentage of Native American residents (8%) of the fifty states. Over two thirds of the state's population–and the largest population of homeless individuals–reside in the Albuquerque metropolitan area. The climate in Albuquerque is that of a high mountain desert, with cold nights and warm days. There is easy access from other large cities to the North and West; the two interstate highways in New Mexico, one oriented North-South, and the second East-West, intersect in the center of Albuquerque.

Characteristics of Homeless Persons in Albuquerque

Homeless persons in Albuquerque have been estimated to number 1,200 to 2,000 persons on any given night and, due to the transient nature of Albuquerque's homeless population, 10,000 to 16,000 different homeless individuals each year (Robertson, 1987). A survey conducted at Albuquerque's Health Care for the Homeless (HCH) Clinic revealed that about 50% of the homeless persons receiving medical services reported a problem with alcohol, and 25% of all persons reported problems with other substance abuse (McMurray-Avila and Hammond, 1987). As in other large cities the majority of homeless persons congregate in the downtown area; other gathering places include the area surrounding the University of New Mexico campus, and the forested banks of the Rio Grande River (bosque), which bisects the city.

Substance Abuse Treatment Services for Homeless Persons

Before the demonstration program began, there were only a few outpatient, and one inpatient, community programs which provided treatment and support services to homeless substance abusers. The only state-funded inpatient alcohol rehabilitation program serving the county has 14 beds for medical detoxification and 26 beds for rehabilitation (21-day program). Homeless persons seeking treatment services, therefore, could receive up to one month of housing before being discharged back onto the streets, where maintaining sobriety is often an insurmountable challenge.

PROJECT H&ART

The NIAAA-funded demonstration program augments existing services by adding essential residential programs for homeless substance abusers in this community. The services thought to be most essential are a residential detoxification program, and a transitional housing, case management, and support services program. Project H&ART (Housing and Alcohol Research Team) is a collaborative effort of three Albuquerque-based organizations. The Lovelace Medical Foundation (LMF), the grantee, contracted with HCH to provide detoxification services, and with St. Martin's Hospitality Center (SMC) to provide rehabilitation and transitional housing services.

Target Population, Procedures, and Client Flow

The targeted population includes homeless adults (ages 18 and over) with alcohol abuse problems, who have been in the Albuquerque area for at least three months. Persons with dependent children, serious mental illnesses, or organic brain syndrome are not eligible for the program. Standardized assessments used in the screening process include questions on alcohol use derived from the Diagnostic and Statistical Manual, Revised Edition (DSM-IIIR) (APA, 1987); and the mini-mental status exam (Folstein et al. 1975). To be eligible, subjects must meet DSM-IIIR criteria for alcohol abuse or dependence (with or without use of other substances), and score 23 or above on the mini-mental status examination.

Clients first learn about Project H&ART from staff at SMC; from the outreach or clinic staff at HCH; or from one of the agencies which provides other services to homeless clients. The project screener, a research staff member, interviews potential clients and determines study eligibility. Eligible persons are asked if they are interested in enrolling in Project

H&ART, and willing to be randomized to one of the three comparison groups. Conditions imposed by the study also are explained at this time. Persons not interested in participating are not excluded from later entry into the study. Those who agree to participate are examined at the HCH clinic by a physician's assistant knowledgeable about health problems of homeless persons, signs of substance abuse, and potential medical complications of alcohol and drug withdrawal. Persons not at significant medical risk are transported to the detoxification facility. If detoxification in a medical inpatient setting is indicated, the client is transported to a state-funded facility for detoxification under medical supervision.

Initial Intervention: The Detoxification Program

The HCH component of Project H&ART provides short-term (two to ten days) alcohol detoxification in a 10-bed, residential facility. The program is designed according to the social model approach (Shaw and Borkman, 1990). This approach, which has been used successfully in other parts of the country, most notably in California, relies on human interaction and support provided by staff and other residents to help peers through the withdrawal process (O'Briant et al., 1977; Sparadeo, 1982; McGovern, 1983). Residents are involved in daily housekeeping activities, on-site groups, and recreation/social activities, and are transported twice a week to Alcoholics Anonymous and Narcotics Anonymous meetings. No medications are administered during the alcohol withdrawal process. The goals of the detoxification program are to provide a warm, home-like environment; to empower residents to seek a "way out," gain self-esteem, and learn self-care; and to assist residents during the physiological process of alcohol withdrawal in a safe, supportive non-medical setting. The staff include a program manager, also a registered nurse, six full-time recovery aides, and a few part-time recovery aides. The majority of these aides are in recovery themselves, and represent a diversity of ethnic/cultural backgrounds, including Native American, Hispanic, non-Hispanic white, and Afro-American.

Those successfully completing detoxification receive a baseline assessment by research staff, are randomly assigned to one of the study groups, and are transported to their residences.

Extended Interventions–Goals, Treatment Rationale and Program Description

Group I. Group I is the high intensity, intervention group in which clients receive case management and substance abuse treatment services, and are provided with alcohol- and drug-free transitional housing, staffed by peer residence managers. The theoretical model for this group is based upon the chemical dependency disease model (Millman, 1988) wherein chemical dependency is thought to be a primary condition, the treatment for which emphasizes the need for abstinence from all mood altering substances. A case management model is utilized in Group I; the four case managers on staff also serve as substance abuse treatment counselors. Twelve-step programs, group processes, and peer support are important components of the treatment intervention. The intervention also incorporates treatment components derived from other addiction treatment models. These include educational and cognitive approaches and behavior modeling (Miller, 1989). This strategy integrates principles and techniques thought to be most effective into a broad-based, comprehensive program. Group I houses up to 30 clients for up to four months. The facility is composed of three, grouped four-plexes located in a low income neighborhood.

The program activities are divided into two, two-month blocks. In the initial block clients are discouraged from looking for jobs, and those with jobs must agree to take a leave of absence or decrease their hours so that they can participate in the program. Since the apartments are not licensed treatment centers, program activities are conducted off-site in a nearby office building. Case managers and other paid and volunteer staff conduct education-oriented groups, and provide group therapy, individual therapy (one to two sessions per week), art therapy, and psychodrama. Recreational events are scheduled weekly. Activities are scheduled from 9 a.m. to 3 p.m. five days a week. Residents also are required to attend weekly community meetings and daily AA or NA meetings, although the monitoring and enforcement of these requirements has varied over the course of the program.

The second two month block is much less structured; case managers encourage clients to acquire jobs, and to develop social and other living skills. Attempts are made at this time to locate services for those who are not able to work or need to be placed in supervised facilities. During this period weekly individual counseling sessions are continued and the clients meet with their counselors on an as-needed basis. Seven residence managers (who are recovering alcoholics/addicts), staff both *the Group I and II residences* and are urged to encourage positive group interactions and peer group support.

Group II. Participants in this medium intensity intervention have less active intervention. They are provided an alcohol- and drug-free living environment, and support from recovering residence managers. Since members of Group II are not assigned case managers, residents are encouraged to develop their own group and peer support networks, and seek treatment for their alcohol and drug abuse on their own initiatives. This approach is based on the expectation that participants, with assistance from peers in recovery (residence managers), will become motivated to develop group support systems within their respective housing units.

Clients in Group II are housed in one of two locations: the first is a two story, eight-plex; the other is a complex of eight, one story apartments. (Four, side-by-side apartments face each other, separated by a courtyard.) One apartment at each site serves as an office and group activities room. The average daily census in Group II ranges from 20 to 30 clients. The only requirements of Group II residents are that they remain alcohol and drug free; attend weekly community meetings; and inform staff twice weekly about services they have received in the community (including job placement, health care, mental health, and substance abuse counseling services).

Group III. Persons assigned to the low intensity comparison group are provided with unsupervised, community-based housing, monitoring of self-initiated treatment services, and they submit to random alcohol and drug testing. Clients are required to complete service utilization forms twice weekly.

The staff spent considerable time discussing relapse issues before enrollment began. After much debate, and after reviewing several options and approaches, the staff decided that the need for maintaining an alcohol/drug free environment in the housing units was paramount. Therefore, clients are not allowed to use alcohol or drugs, either at the housing sites or elsewhere. Relapse results in removal from housing. Although this seems harsh, the team was reinforced in their decision when the clients themselves voted to support this policy. Clients are required to submit to breath tests, for alcohol content, and urine tests, for detection of other drug use. Such monitoring is performed randomly by a designated staff person who does not have other program responsibilities. Monitoring is also performed by any staff member if the client is suspected to be using alcohol or drugs (reports by landlords of drug or alcohol use, alcohol odor on breath, unusual behavior).

A special program and research emphasis is on structuring the program to meet the needs of all members of the population, including Hispanics and Native Americans. Ethnicity has emerged as a major factor in defining patterns of alcohol use. Mexican Americans have been found to have a higher incidence of alcohol-related problems than the general population (Gilbert and Cervantes, 1987). Yet there are limited data available about this group's use of alcohol, or about the special treatment needs for homeless Hispanic persons. The same holds true for Native Americans, who are a high risk group for substance abuse. In one study Native Americans had the highest rate of alcohol abuse among homeless persons (Wright, 1987).

Research Design

The study is a prospective, randomized comparison of three intervention strategies for assisting homeless persons with alcohol-related problems. Participants are randomized to one of the three intervention groups described above. Client interviews are conducted by research staff upon entry into the study, and at four- and ten-month intervals after detoxification. Outcome measures include clients' use of substances of abuse, residential stability, employment stability, level of depression, and measures of self-esteem and self-perception.

The research design also includes a process evaluation, with formative and qualitative components. The formative component includes service documentation, client service utilization monitoring, and a quality assurance program. The types and quantity of case management and residence manager services are entered onto a computerized database and reviewed regularly, as are drop-out rates and reasons clients left the program. These data are analyzed by gender and ethnicity, and assist program staff in redirecting intervention efforts to increase program effectiveness. Program implementation is monitored to ensure that the interventions are implemented as planned.

The qualitative component consists of approximately 100 client and staff interviews, conducted by an anthropologist. Focused interviews collect information regarding the day-to-day functioning of the treatment program; assess the program's strengths and weaknesses; compare and contrast the three intervention programs; assess the elements of the programs which were most important to clients in helping them effect life-style changes; and assess whether client perceptions of the program vary by gender and ethnic background.

PROGRAM START-UP ISSUES

The implementation of new programs within a six month period was a challenge to the three participating agencies. Since historically so few services had been provided to homeless persons in New Mexico, the pool of persons in the community who had experience managing or staffing programs such as those envisioned was very small. The start-up needs were great: a large staff needed to be hired and trained, and facilities acquired and furnished. Several difficulties, described below, were encountered. Nevertheless, the start-up phase, which began in October, 1990, was completed by mid-April, 1991, and the first client was enrolled into Project H&ART on April 23, 1991.

Several implementation issues arose during the start-up period of HCH's detoxification program pertaining to: zoning; staffing/training; and staff acceptance of the social model approach to detoxifying clients. As with most cities, the zoning ordinances in Albuquerque discourage the development of residential substance abuse programs. HCH had purchased–and was ready to renovate–two adjacent, four-bedroom duplexes in the North Valley of Albuquerque. Although the necessary conditional use permit was initially denied based on neighborhood opposition, the denial was overturned upon subsequent appeal and the permit was obtained. The delay in obtaining the permit resulted, however, in the need to utilize a temporary location for detoxification services (from April to August, 1991). The physical environment of this temporary site (several small, two-bedroom apartments) necessitated using one apartment as a community living space and the use of one of the bedrooms as a communal dining area. As program beds were filled, space became a limiting factor, and meetings often were moved outside onto the lawn, as weather permitted. In September, 1991, HCH began operating its program out of the permanent residences.

One advantage to the delay in program start-up was the opportunity to spend significant time in staff development and training. Staff development activities ranged from participation in a Navajo healing ceremony to NIAAA-funded technical assistance and staff training by an expert in social model programs.

There was strong support from HCH administration and the new program staff for the development of a social model approach to detoxification. However, the existing HCH medical staff had not been involved in designing this program and did not fully understand nor trust the model. This led to some initial resistance from the medical staff involved in physical examinations and triage. Since there was little trust in the beginning that clients could be detoxified safely without medical personnel on-site and without medications, there was disagreement over which clients needed to be referred elsewhere for medical detoxification and which should be admitted to the residential program. This was eventually resolved by hiring an additional staff member–a physician's assistant–who had extensive experience working with alcoholics in detoxification, and less apprehension regarding the social model approach.

The transitional housing program also experienced some difficulties during start-up. Procuring appropriate housing leases and staffing the residences proved to be major hurdles during the project's initiation. According to the Wittman (1989) model, the most favorable housing environment for residential programs incorporates a centralized community cooking and dining area design, with all residents of an intervention group living under one roof. While the potential of this design for facilitating group cohesiveness was recognized, program staff were unsuccessful in locating and leasing residences with this type of environment, due to minimal availability and prohibitive cost. Therefore, participants were housed in two-bedroom, apartment buildings (Groups I and II), motel rooms and single residence units (Group III).

During the process of securing apartment leases for housing clients and hiring program staff, the original experimental design underwent some changes. In the original proposal, for example, resident managers were to be live-in staff who received, as part of their salaries, rent-free apartments. The rationale was that there would be an abundance of men and women in recovery (with at least one year of sobriety) willing to work under these conditions. However, attempts to recruit and hire recovering individuals as resident managers at the budgeted salary levels were unsuccessful. Program managers, therefore, were forced to abandon the live-in requirement, opting instead to fill these positions with shift workers. The positions changed from "resident managers" to "residence managers."

The most troublesome problem was the difficulty maintaining the integrity of Group III. Without supervision, alcohol and drug use became a significant problem among the Group III clients. There were several incidents in which multiple homeless friends were invited to move into the Group III residences. Property was damaged and stolen, and landlords began refusing to continue renting apartments to SMC. Problems in administering this part of the program led to many changes in housing locations. Client housing shifted from well-kept, single residence units to seedy motel rooms equipped with small stoves and refrigerators, to two-bedroom apartments. It became apparent that the safety of clients and staff could not be assured. Finally, in December, 1991, after 92 persons were randomized to Group III, housing for members of this group was discontinued and a fourth group, a non-housed control group, replaced the original Group III. Although this change was welcomed by the SMC staff who administered Group III, reaction of HCH staff to the situation that one-third of the persons entering the study would not receive housing was quite negative; indeed, some staff threatened to resign. After a great deal of discussion it was agreed that women would be randomized only to Groups I and II. It was further agreed that men assigned to the non-housed group would be counseled by a staff person before discharge from the detoxification program, and would be referred to other available services.

The major challenge to the research program was maintaining the integrity of the research design while maintaining a sense of collaboration and teamwork with program staff. The project's management staff spent a considerable amount of time attempting to integrate the research and program needs of the project. A management team composed of the Principal Investigator, the Executive Directors of the two subcontracting agencies, and the program managers of the three agencies was formed. This team meets weekly or biweekly to discuss programmatic, logistic, and psychological issues involved in implementing the demonstration program. An example of one successful start-up project initiated by the management team was Project H&ART's version of a "dress rehearsal," conducted the week before enrollment was to begin. During this rehearsal some staff role-played clients and "acted out" all stages of the process (from initial screening at the day shelter, to the physical examination, detoxification, testing, randomization, and program intake). Other staff played themselves and performed anticipated job duties. This exercise proved beneficial, not only because logistical problems were uncovered that needed resolution, but because it promoted good relationships among team members, and gave staff an appreciation of the client's perspective. The team building efforts of the management team worked well for the project. For the most part, problems were addressed as they arose, and most individuals contributed to the solutions.

The three program managers also met weekly to coordinate activities, solve problems, and exchange information. Most issues were resolved at this level. Finally, staff retreats and lunches were held, which fostered team building and boosted morale. All of these efforts resulted in fairly strong cohesion, and maximized communications among all staff members.

CHARACTERISTICS OF PARTICIPANTS

During Project H&ART's enrollment period (April 1991-August 31, 1992), 980 potential clients were contacted. Of those, 665 (68%) were screened and found to meet the eligibility criteria described earlier. One hundred and one individuals did not provide sufficient information at screening, and were thus ineligible. Of the remaining 214 persons who did not meet eligibility criteria, 15% were found to have a significant mental illness, 19% were not alcohol abusers, 30% did not meet the three month residency requirement, 7% had family members requiring support, 2%

were not homeless, .5% were under age, .5% had pending court dates, 13% had personal issues, and 13% were ineligible for other reasons such as: job, not interested, or violent behavior. Of the 665 persons who were eligible, 498 (75%) entered the detoxification program (2 of these were first triaged to the state-funded medical detoxification program), and only 29 persons (6%) left before successfully completing detoxification.

A modified version of the Alcohol Withdrawal Assessment Scale (Naranjo and Sellers, 1986) was used to evaluate and monitor withdrawal symptoms experienced by clients. Every client who remained in the program for at least one day was assessed for symptoms of alcohol or other drug withdrawal. Those with symptoms were monitored regularly. Three hundred twenty-two (67%) of these individuals had no symptoms of alcohol or drug withdrawal. None of the clients experienced seizures and only one individual had symptoms that were serious enough to warrant transportation to a medical facility.

One hundred sixty-one participants (34% of those who completed the detoxification program) were randomized to Group I; 164 (35%) to Group II; 92 (20%) to Group III; and 52 (11%) to the non-housed control Group IV. Client ages ranged from 18 to 67, with a median age of 37 years (Table 1).

The definition of homelessness for Project H&ART clients included not only those staying in shelters, and living on the streets and in abandoned buildings, but also those who were marginally housed (those who were living in "doubled up" situations and other persons whose entry into the program may have prevented them from becoming homeless). Clients varied in the degree of chronicity of homelessness (Table 1).

As of September, 1992, the drop out rate from all three intervention groups was 75% (a total of 282 of 378 subjects assigned to Groups I-III). Dropout rates were similar for the three housed intervention groups: 71% for Group I; 82% for Group II; and 70% for Group III clients (Chi-square, 8.02, p = .53). However, there was a significant difference in the reasons clients left the program (Table 2). In Group I, the largest percentage of dropouts left on their own accord without identifying a specific reason. In Groups II and III, however, chemical use was the reason for discharge for the majority of clients who left the program.

DISCUSSION

Results of the baseline interviews indicated that clients entering Project H&ART were from the population that the demonstration program had intended to reach–almost all were primary alcohol abusers who had been homeless or were in danger of becoming homeless. There were several

Table 1. Characteristics of the 469 Project H&ART Participants

Variable	N	%
Gender		
Males	413	88.1
Females	56	11.9
Race/Ethnicity		
Non-Hispanic White	196	41.8
Hispanic	146	31.1
Native American	80	17.1
Other	47	10.0
Age (Median = 37)		
18-29	92	19.8
30-44	268	57.6
45 and over	109	22.6
Employment Status		
Full-time employment previous 12 months	112	23.9
Part-time or seasonal employment previous 12 months	113	24.1
Unemployed previous 12 months	229	48.8
Other(student, retired, military, etc.)	15	3.2
Primary Substance of Abuse (Self-reports)		
alcohol	437	93.2
cocaine	16	3.4
heroin	7	1.5
other*	8	1.7
no drug/alcohol problem	1	0.2
Years of Homelessness-Lifetime		
Never homeless	11	2.3
Homeless <1 year	164	35.0
Homeless 1-4 years	179	38.2
Homeless 5-10 years	68	14.5
Homeless > 10 years	40	8.5
Indeterminable	7	1.5

*sedatives, cannabis, hallucinogens, inhalants, methodone

Table 2.   Drop-outs by Housed Intervention Group & Reason, for Participants enrolling in Project H&ART by 31 May 1992*

	Left On Own Accord		Discharged- Chemical Use		Discharged- Other rule Violations		Other**	
	N	%	N	%	N	%	N	%
Group I	54	52.9	29	28.4	18	17.7	1	1.0
GROUP II	32	27.6	54	46.6	28	24.1	2	1.7
GROUP III	22	34.4	35	54.7	7	10.9	0	0.0

*Fisher's exact test comparing drop-out rates by group was 21.71. p = .0014.
**This category includes institutionalized and deceased individuals.

unexpected developments, however, in the implementation of Project H&ART. The first set of unexpected findings related to the characteristics of the population entering the program. First, clients generally were younger than anticipated. Staff's perceptions were that most would be men over age fifty who were chronically homeless. In fact, only 16 (3%) of the clients were at least 50 years old and had been homeless for five years or more.

This may in large part reflect the changing nature of homeless populations in this country. Homelessness now affects a broad cross-section of the population (Rossi, 1989), and studies increasingly portray the homeless population as younger, and more heterogeneous than the skid row populations previously described, and include a greater proportion of minorities and women (Fischer and Breakey, 1991). It is also clear that the program did not successfully attract some members of the targeted population. Outreach workers at HCH reported on several occasions that they had repeatedly approached certain elderly, homeless gentlemen in futile efforts to convince them to enter the program.

Another unanticipated development was the enrollment of fewer women than expected. It is not clear whether the smaller than expected number of women enrolling in the program was due to an initial overestimate of the number of single homeless women in the community, or to a reluctance by women to enter a program that included both genders. It is well-known that women who are homeless–especially those who are substance abusers–often have been victimized, physically and sexually (Bassuk and Rosenberg, 1988; D'Ercole and Struening, 1990). These women understandably may have had reservations about entering Project H&ART, with its predominantly male staff and clients.

Other unexpected findings became evident when clients entered the detoxification program. First, very few clients were triaged to the state-funded medical detoxification facility. Second, staff discovered that the majority of persons entering the detoxification program did not need detoxification services. The majority experienced no symptoms of withdrawal. Those who did experience symptoms had a lower than anticipated incidence of medical problems during detoxification. Finally, the drop-out rate from the detoxification program was much lower than the anticipated rate of 25%; 94% of persons completed the program and were randomized to the transitional housing program.

Lessons also were learned regarding the approach to zoning issues. It is well known that programs must anticipate neighborhood resistance to the establishment of treatment programs and that there is a need for ongoing education and relationship-building in the community (Rubenstein et al., 1991). The Albuquerque team found that these efforts must be inherent to the program. The detoxification program has sponsored several community meetings and picnics, and staff members have picked up litter in the neighborhood, painted over graffiti, and plan to shovel walkways this winter. Staff investments of energy, time, and creative brainstorming have had mixed results, however. Local resistance to the detoxification program has waxed and waned over the past year, but a great deal of the resentment and fear has been quelled through the efforts of program staff.

The program has experienced several barriers to implementing the planned research design. The most significant of these was the necessity to discontinue the housing component of Group III. This design change caused several problems. There was a negative reaction by some staff, who felt that it was unfair to provide for only two-thirds of the clients. Also the discontinuation of housing for Group III clients appeared to have a negative impact on client recruitment. Finally, this change split the comparison population into two groups, with smaller sample sizes. Group III has 92 clients, and Group IV, 52 clients.

In conclusion, the project was implemented as designed, although complications due to zoning restrictions, the availability of housing sites, and difficulties recruiting staff necessitated some start-up delays and program modifications. The most significant program modification was the discontinuation of housing for Group III clients. Lessons have been learned regarding the characteristics of persons who are willing to enter a research demonstration program, the need for detoxification services in programs of this kind, and the need to establish good relationships and communications among service and research staff. Preliminary results indicate that the majority of clients dropped out of the program before their four month period of housing ended. Follow-up studies will determine what may have precipitated clients' departure from Project H&ART, and the characteristics of clients who manage to sustain a personal program of recovery.

REFERENCES

American Psychiatric Association (1987). *The third diagnostic and statistical manual of mental disorders* (Rev. ed.). Washington, DC: Author.

Bassuk, E. L., & Rosenberg, L. (1988). "Why does family homelessness occur?" *American Journal of Public Health, 78*:783-788.

D'Ercole, A., & Struening, E. (1990 April). "Victimization among homeless women: Implications for service delivery." *Journal of Community Psychology, 18*:141-152.

Fischer, P. J., & Breakey, W. R. (1991). "The epidemiology of alcohol, drug, and mental disorders among homeless persons." *American Psychologist, 46*(11):1115-1128.

Folstein, M. F., Folstein, P. R., & McHugh, P. R. (1975). "Mini-mental state: A practical guide for grading the cognitive state of patients for the clinician." *Journal of Psychiatric Research, 12*:189-198.

Gilbert, M. J., & Cervantes, R. C. (1987). Mexican Americans and alcohol. *Monographs of the Spanish Speaking Mental Health Research Center, 11*.

McGovern, M. P. (1983). "Comparative evaluation of medical versus social treatment of alcohol withdrawal syndrome." *Journal of Clinical Psychology, 39*:791-803.

McMurray-Avila, M., & Hammond, R. (1987). Results of mental health screening study among homeless adults. Health Care for the Homeless, Albuquerque, N.M. 87102, (unpublished report).

Miller, W. R., & Hester, R. K. (1989). "Treating alcohol problems: Toward an informed eclecticism." In: *Handbook of Alcoholism Treatment and Approaches*, Hesker, R. K. & Miller, W. R. (Eds.). Pergamon Press, N.Y.

Millman, R. B. (1988). "Evaluation and clinical management of cocaine abusers." *Journal of Clinical Psychiatry, 40* (Suppl. 2):27-33.

Naranjo, C. A., & Sellers, E. M. (1986). "Clinical assessment and pharmacotherapy of the alcohol withdrawal syndrome." In: Galanter, M. (Ed.), *Recent developments in alcoholism*. New York: Plenum Press, pp. 265-281.

O'Briant, R., Petersen, N. W., & Heacock, D. "How safe is social setting detoxification?" *Alcohol Health and Research World*, Winter 1976/1977, *1*(2):22-27.

Robertson, M. (1987). "Report on homelessness in Albuquerque." Albuquerque Department of Health and Human Services, Albuquerque, N.M., 87102.

Rossi, P. (1989). *"Down and out in America."* Chicago: University of Chicago Press.

Rubenstein, L., Osterloh, K., Hancock, P. & Russau, B. (1991). "Overcoming

NIMBY ("Not in My Back Yard") issues," Housing Initiatives for Homeless People with Alcohol and other Drug Problems: Proceedings of a National Conference, National Institute on Alcohol Abuse and Alcoholism, 71-77.

Shaw, S. & Borkman, T. (1990). *Social model alcohol recovery: An environmental approach.* Bridge Focus, Inc., Burbank, CA.

Sparadeo, F. R. (1982). "Evaluation of a social-setting detoxification program." *Journal of Studies on Alcohol, 43*:1124-1136.

U.S. Bureau of the Census, 1990 Census, New Mexico.

Wittman, F.D. (1989). "Housing models for alcohol programs serving homeless people." *Contemporary Drug Problems, 16*:483-504.

Wright, J. D., Knight, J. W., Weber-Burdin, E., & Lam, J. (1987). "Ailments and alcohol-health status among the drinking homeless." *Alcohol Health Research World, 11*:22-27.

Case Managed Residential Care for Homeless Addicted Veterans: Evanston/VA

Annie R. Pope, MSW, ACSW
Kendon J. Conrad, PhD
William Baxter, MSSW
Phillip Elbaum, MSW
Joseph Lisiecki, MA
Amin Daghestani, MD
Cheryl Hultman, PhD
John Lyons, PhD

SUMMARY. The Case Managed Residential Care (CMRC) program, a social rehabilitation model, was implemented in a traditional medical environment as a response to the needs of homeless chem-

Annie R. Pope, William Baxter, Phillip Elbaum, Joseph Lisiecki and Amin Daghestani are affiliated with Edward Hines, Jr. VA Hospital, Hines IL 60141. Kendon J. Conrad, Cheryl Hultman, and John Lyons are affiliated with the Center for Health Services and Policy Research, Northwestern University, 629 Noyes Street, Evanston IL 60208.

Address correspondence to: Annie R. Pope, Chief, Social Work Service, Hines VA Hospital, Hines IL 60141.

This research demonstration project is supported by: (1) a National Institute on Alcohol Abuse and Alcoholism grant (AA08818); (2) Hines VA Hospital for use of the physical plant and hospital customary services; (3) VA Department of Mental Health and Behavioral Sciences for renovation funds; and (4) the VA Midwest Health Services Research and Development Field Program.

[Haworth co-indexing entry note]: "Case Managed Residential Care for Homeless Addicted Veterans: Evanston/VA." Pope, Annie R. et al. Co-published simultaneously in the *Alcoholism Treatment Quarterly* (The Haworth Press, Inc.) Vol. 10, No. 3/4, 1993, pp. 155-169; and: *Treatment of the Chemically Dependent Homeless: Theory and Implementation in Fourteen American Projects* (ed: Kendon J. Conrad, Cheryl I. Hultman, and John S. Lyons) The Haworth Press, Inc., 1993, pp. 155-169. Multiple copies of this article/chapter may be purchased from The Haworth Document Delivery Center [1-800-3-HAWORTH: 9:00 a.m. - 5:00 p.m. (EST)].

cally dependent veterans, many of whom were also mentally ill. These veterans were resistant to traditional interventions and were frequently rejected or discharged prematurely by many community resources due to the facilities' inability to manage them and/or the veterans inability or unwillingness to participate. This paper describes the target population, the objectives of the research demonstration studying the experimental and customary treatments, and the theoretical foundations of treatment. Then it describes some of the key, practical issues involved in implementing the CMRC and draws implications useful for the treatment of this needy and underserved population.

The Case Managed Residential Care for Homeless Addicted Veterans Research project, a joint project of the Center for Health Services and Policy Research of Northwestern University in Evanston, Illinois and the Edward Hines, Jr. VA Hospital, is the only NIAAA Cooperative Agreement project which specifically targets homeless veterans with substance abuse problems. The project's clinical component is located at Hines VA Hospital in the Social Work and Psychiatry Services. Hines VAH is the fifth largest in the VA system of 171 hospitals with over 1,100 beds. The research component is coordinated through the Center for Health Services and Policy Research (CHSPR) at Northwestern University. Established in 1977, the center includes a multidisciplinary research staff with expertise in program evaluation, policy analysis, organizational behavior, health economics and quality improvement. The research staff is hired by Northwestern University and is located at the Midwest Health Services Research and Development (HSR&D) Field Program at Hines VAH. The collaboration in health services research between CHSPR and HSR&D is longstanding and extends to the inception of the HSR&D Field Program in 1983.

BACKGROUND

Research on substance abuse treatment is considered a high priority by the Department of Veterans Affairs (VA) since the impact of substance abuse on the VA is enormous. For example, in 1989, the estimated cost of VA inpatient and outpatient care for veterans with substance abuse problems was more than $1.7 billion (Moos, Swindle, and Pasch, 1991). The research conducted on these substance abuse patients demonstrated a recidivism rate of 36% at six months and 43% at one year following their index admission.

The VA substance abuse patients generally present with more than a substance abuse disorder. Of the veterans represented in the Moos et al. study (1992), 48% had a dual diagnosis of substance abuse and a psychiatric disorder, 24% had a multiple diagnosis of two or more psychiatric disorders along with their substance abuse disorder and 67% had a physical (medical) diagnosis as well as a substance abuse disorder.

The Case Managed Residential Care (CMRC) facility utilizes a social model program implemented in a traditional medical environment. The program targets homeless, chemically dependent veterans, a third of whom are also mentally ill. These veterans are resistant to traditional interventions and often fit the "revolving door" definition of recidivism in both inpatient and community treatment programs. They are frequently rejected or discharged prematurely by many community resources due to the facilities' inability to manage them and/or the veterans' inability or unwillingness to deal with the structure of a substance abuse treatment program.

OBJECTIVES OF THE PROJECT

In a randomized controlled trial, the project is testing the effectiveness of the CMRC in comparison to a control group receiving customary care. The goals of the CMRC are to: (1) increase the length of time engaged in treatment; (2) reduce alcohol/drug use and extend periods of recovery from substance abuse disorders; (3) improve vocational/economic status; and, (4) improve mental health status.

Treatment Population

Subjects were selected based on the following criteria: (1) male, since only about 1% of this VA population are female, (2) inpatient on a Hines VA substance abuse or psychiatric unit, (3) homeless one month prior to admission, (4) active substance abuse diagnosis, (5) plans to live within a 99 mile radius of Hines VAH, (6) medically and psychiatrically stable, (7) no history of violent behavior in the last three years, (8) no active warrants or impending incarceration, and (9) no neurological impairment. The presence of other psychiatric disorders did not result in exclusion.

The following description of the treatment population is based on data obtained from the initial 201 of the planned 270 subjects who have been randomized into the study. The subjects averaged 41 years of age, 12.6 years of education, and 71% were black. Twenty-one percent were skilled manual laborers, 38% were semi-skilled workers, and about 20% were unskilled. Approximately 50% were unemployed in the past year. Nearly two-thirds were unemployed in the past 30 days. The average lifetime use of alcohol to the point of intoxication was 15.2 years. The average use of other drugs was 12.2 years. Thirty-four percent reported that they had previously been in inpatient psychiatric treatment.

The subjects reported at baseline that of the 60 nights prior to their current hospital admission, 47% had been spent in shelters, subways or buses, abandoned buildings, cars, outdoor public places, drug houses and other undomiciled arrangements. Another 26% of the previous nights had been spent in emergency shelters, transitional housing, hotels or motels, single room occupancy apartments (SRO) or boarding houses. About 10% of the nights had been spent in alcohol and drug free facilities, hospitals, nursing homes, residential treatment facilities, or jails. Approximately 9% of the nights had been spent temporarily in a parent or guardian's apartment or house and about 2% in their own apartment or house. The remaining 6% of the nights were unaccounted for or could not be remembered.

The most common primary substance abuse problem with this population is cocaine (46.4%) followed by alcohol (42.5%) and heroin (10.3%). The majority (64%) have problems with two or more substances. The most common secondary substances of abuse are alcohol (31%), cocaine (19%) and heroin (7%). From the above mentioned statistics, it is apparent that we succeeded in enrolling the intended population of homeless, alcohol and drug dependent veterans, about a third of whom are also mentally ill. Among homeless veterans, this is probably the major subgroup that is the most difficult to treat. In our experience, relationships are often difficult to establish with this client population. Residents frequently feel alienated by health care providers and society. Many residents have severe characterological problems and have become estranged from their social support system.

The Setting of Customary Care

The Hines VA Hospital Psychiatry Service is comprised of three 30-bed inpatient substance abuse units and three 30-bed psychiatry units. Additionally, each program has a large outpatient treatment clinic. Each substance abuse treatment inpatient unit is organized according to a medical model, staffed primarily by 14 registered nurses, 1.5 physicians, 2 substance abuse counselors and 1 masters level social worker with access to psychologists, dieticians, kinesio, vocational, educational, occupational and recreational therapists. Although patients may stay up to 21 days, the average length of stay in the inpatient substance abuse treatment units is 17 days.

During the hospital stay in customary care, patients receive substance abuse and abstinence education, individual and group therapy. They participate in various rehabilitation medicine activities. Inpatients are evaluated by a physician and treated for any coexisting medical and/or psychiatric conditions. Patients are seen by a social worker for assessment, psychotherapy and discharge planning. Discharge placement referrals are made to halfway houses, financial, legal, mental health clinics, family service agencies and self-help resources within the VA and community. Many of the community halfway houses that customary care patients are referred to have purchase of care contracts with the VA By our definition customary care includes, not just the 21 day hospital program, but also all other services received over the one year period of observation in the study.

Theory of Treatment–Customary Care

Customary care on inpatient substance abuse treatment units provides a structured, therapeutic approach to acutely ill patients. It provides the necessary medical and psychiatric resources to manage the acute phase of each patient's illness. The goal of customary care is to detoxify patients from alcohol and other drugs, stabilize their medical and psychiatric conditions and prepare them for continuing outpatient care. In essence, the goal of customary care is to introduce the patient to recovery and a drug free lifestyle. Interventions focus on pharmacological therapy, individual, group and family therapies and a strong emphasis on 12-step self-help recovery groups, e.g., Alcoholics Anonymous and Narcotics Anonymous. The strengths of customary care include: (1) ability to provide intensive medical, psychiatric and psychosocial interventions in a highly structured setting; and (2) easy access to comprehensive hospital-wide services.

The major weaknesses of customary care are: (1) the inpatient intervention is brief, particularly considering the complex nature of these patients; (2) high cost of treatment due to the many highly specialized resources used to provide inpatient care; and (3) being institutionally-based, the staff is limited from becoming involved with patients in the community.

After discharge from the 21 day inpatient program, customary care within VA provides a range of diverse, often highly specialized, services. For the person who is psychiatrically impaired due to mental illness and/or substance abuse and who has a variety of psychosocial problems, this fragmentation of services can interact with the patient's fears, cognitive deficits, feelings of being overwhelmed and low frustration tolerance to produce non-compliance with treatment. Customary care provides in-office therapy which depends on the client sustaining sufficient motivation and mental organization to keep scheduled weekly appointments in an initially unfamiliar agency. Customary care does not appear to be particularly effective for this population. Existing programs often lack staffing to provide follow up and support to the client that would insure proper aftercare and treatment compliance.

The Setting of CMRC Program

The CMRC is a 30-bed facility on the hospital grounds. The expected length of stay is 3 to 6 months. The CMRC is staffed with 3 masters level social workers who function as case managers, 1.5 food service personnel, 1 program coordinator, 1 program assistant, 1 vocational rehabilitation therapist and 7.5 substance abuse counselors. The ratio of residents to case managers in the CMRC residency phase is 10:1, while this ratio increases to about 25:1 in the community follow up phase. A number of the staff are recovering persons. The clinical staff is supported by the Chief, Social Work Service, and two supervisory social workers assigned to Psychiatry Service, and a staff psychiatrist.

Theory of Treatment–CMRC

CMRC treatment focuses on here and now issues. A cognitive, behavioral, problem-solving approach is used in contrast to traditional intrapsychic models. These intrapsychic models often deal with early life experiences and antecedents of problematic behavior, and are not always relevant to the practical issues of daily living. Relapse prevention skills training is an essential component of CMRC treatment consisting of assertive drink and drug refusal, coping with relapse, social networking and anger management. Self-help groups are emphasized for emotional support and to enhance coping behavior in addition to maintaining abstinence.

Clinical studies indicate that dually diagnosed individuals are strongly predisposed to homelessness because their substance abuse leads to disruptive behavior and cognitive impairments (Castaneda, 1992). Housing and vocational counseling are essential for this population in order to continue their new coping skills and abstinence. For the dually diagnosed, the management of psychotropic medications and the monitoring of mental status is essential since many dually diagnosed persons use drugs as self-medication.

Benefits of the case management model. Case management is designed to help residents to overcome barriers to attaining self-care and self-sufficiency. It should facilitate empowerment and improve self-esteem. Empowerment refers to the development of skills that enable a person to implement interpersonal influence, improve role performance, and develop an effective support system, in other words, to help clients take control of their lives (Thompson, Anderson and Boeringa, 1992). The residents are expected to achieve a sense of security, resourcefulness and self-actualization. The case management model is anticipated to integrate the clinical and the environmental interventions into one service delivery system. This model, as adapted, should reduce factors contributing to non-compliance with treatment.

Description of the CMRC Program

Detoxification and stabilization. The CMRC program can be described in four phases. Phase one includes a five to ten day medical detoxification on psychiatry or substance abuse treatment units as previously described under "customary care." During that period, veterans are screened by inpatient social workers for participation in the study. Randomization occurs after the study is explained by a research assistant and the veteran has signed the informed consent to participate. After randomization, all control subjects continue receiving customary treatment as described earlier.

CMRC subjects are discharged from the hospital to the CMRC as soon as they are medically stable, usually after five to ten days. CMRC case managers coordinate and collaborate with the inpatient staff to facilitate the transition of inpatients to CMRC. This coordination of the transition by the assigned case manager initiates the therapeutic relationship.

Orientation, assessment, and planning. Phase two is the beginning of case managed residential care utilizing the case management model (Kanter, 1989). The first two weeks are devoted to an orientation which is coordinated by the case manager who is assisted by the substance abuse counselors, a vocational rehabilitation therapist and food service manager. These staff collaborate with the resident to develop a comprehensive assessment and treatment plan, thus beginning a process of empowering the resident to manage his own recovery. Significant to this phase is the relationship development that assists residents in becoming empowered, goal focused and realistic regarding their substance abuse. The residents also participate in goal setting for abstinence, employment or other means of financial support, housing and use of leisure time. Although efforts are made to insure each resident's sense of control over his recovery, the CMRC also maintains considerable structure both to insure an environment of abstinence and to be equitable to all residents. Expectations are communicated for residing in the facility and the resident is given a copy of the "Resident's Handbook."

Services provided at the facility such as psychoeducational groups, individual and group therapy, self-help groups and activities of daily living are introduced. Appointments for follow-up visits to outpatient clinics and other community resources are either reviewed or planned. Policy for requesting passes and procedures for alcohol and drug screening are also reviewed.

Continuous assessment and treatment. Phase three is focused on continuous assessment and treatment in the residential setting. It includes planning, engaging and monitoring treatment goals and activities with an emphasis on reintegration into the community. This phase also focuses on maintaining abstinence and initiating community linkages for employment and housing. An effort is made to improve residents' psychosocial skills in multiple areas of their lives, such as resolving family conflicts, job readiness and employment search, use of leisure time, stress management, and relapse prevention. CMRC staff actively engage in identifying community resources for a broad range of services that address identified needs. Staff develop relationships with community service providers for employment, low income housing, substance abuse evaluation, remedial education, and driver's license reinstatement.

Searching for appropriate, longer term housing is critical at this point because it is in this phase that the resident is expected to become more self-sufficient. This phase features intermittent individual psychotherapy where the case managers schedule individual sessions with the residents and are available to meet with them at other times as needed. In individual treatment, focus is directed toward enhancing self esteem and identifying high risk behaviors and stressors that precipitate relapse. These sessions are supplemented by participation in group therapy where networking and problem solving strategies are identified and practiced. Practical issues such as personal money management, budgeting, and reinstatement of credit ratings are addressed. Besides spending individual time with their case managers and substance abuse counselors, residents have group recovery education, social skills training classes and 12-step recovery groups in CMRC. Residents also participate in community 12-step groups.

Since residents experience many crisis situations, continuous monitoring of their behavior and needs is central to therapeutic effectiveness. Psychiatric decompensation and substance abuse relapse are two examples of crisis situations. In the CMRC, when residents decompensate they are assessed and accompanied to the emergency room for evaluation. Frequently, these residents are hospitalized. An important aspect of monitoring is routine, random testing for the use of alcohol and non-prescribed drugs. In CMRC this consists of an alcohol breathalyzer test at the completion of passes exceeding 4 hours. Routine urine specimens are usually also collected after an overnight pass.

The vocational rehabilitation therapist, in concert with other staff, monitors each resident's progress in improving job readiness skills, obtaining training and/or employment. Residents use a computer station for resumes and cover letters. Video cassettes with accompanying workbooks are provided to improve vocational skills and job readiness.

Discharge planning and community case management. Phase four is marked by the resident's discharge to the community and aftercare. The case manager, as a coordinator in the discharge process, establishes a schedule for the remainder of the one year period from the resident's CMRC admission. During this period of follow-up, case management services continue to be provided to assist with community adjustment and problem resolution. This ongoing involvement provides an opportunity to reinforce positive behavior, encourage continued recovery, assist with problem solving and evaluate treatment effectiveness. Clients are seen in the community as well as in the facility. They are actively encouraged to return on an intermittent basis for individual case management and alumni groups. Continued involvement with community 12-step programs is also encouraged.

Theory Gaps

Consensus has yet to be reached regarding the clinical and cost effectiveness of the case management model for persons with substance abuse disorders. The intervention strategy has to demonstrate that reducing recidivism and substance abuse while improving employability, residential stability and positive leisure utilization are possible. In particular, Goering and others have questioned the reduction of recidivism and cost effectiveness of this model (1988). In addition, the philosophy of advocacy inherent in case management intervention can be at odds with the emphasis on empowerment and personal responsibility thought to be critical to recovery.

Discussions with residents have revealed several factors that lead them to accept treatment: (1) personal commitment to abstinence; (2) learning the 12-step program, attending meetings and obtaining sponsors; (3) tired of being helpless and homeless with feelings of hopelessness; (4) growth of self-esteem as a result of interactions with program staff and community experiences; (5) development of meaningful relationships with staff and other residents that allow for bonding experiences; (6) clear communication of expectations and roles; (7) available time to develop and work on goals with opportunities for practice; (8) medication access and compliance; (9) realistic self-appraisal including the ability to examine internal feeling and interactional patterns, and; (10) motivation to embrace a drug free lifestyle with a higher level of functioning.

Clinical staff continue to try to understand the reasons for rejection of treatment interventions. Just as there are residents motivated for change, many others do not choose a more constructive way of life. A small percentage of residents (< 10%) randomized to CMRC do not even reach the CMRC facility. They choose to return to the community, avoiding contact with CMRC for reasons not expressed. Another segment of the population is discharged from inpatient status due to relapse. Some CMRC residents are unable to engage in meaningful relationships. They continue with ambivalence regarding their problems, exhibiting antisocial, fearful, or distrusting behavior. There are others who do not conform to a structured, community group living environment and leave CMRC after a brief stay.

Relapse among substance abusers is a common phenomenon. It occurs for veterans in customary care and those admitted to CMRC. In the customary care program, veterans who relapse are immediately discharged from the hospital. Relapse in CMRC is treated as an opportunity for learning rather than failure. A resident is allowed one relapse and is helped to identify the cognitive and environmental triggers that led to the relapse. He is assisted in developing a relapse prevention plan. Even when residents are administratively discharged for relapse, aftercare services continue to be available from the case manager in the community.

Initially, a high rate of relapse (approximately 30% of all residents during the first eight months of the program) was perceived by staff to be influenced by the CMRC pass policy. To address this issue, a Total Quality Improvement (TQI) approach was applied. TQI, also known as (Total Quality Management), is a systematic approach to productivity improvement using objective methods involving all employees to continuously improve the quality of all products and services (McAdams, 1991). Data were gathered, analyzed and used to make changes in pass policy. The pass policy was changed from a one to a two week restriction in the facility. After two weeks, residents were eligible for passes on a graduated scale. After five weekends, a resident would become eligible for a 48-hour pass. This change in policy has significantly decreased the rate of relapse. As a result of this TQI process, staff felt a sense of empowerment and ownership for the improved and effective operation which appears to have also improved resident outcomes.

Figure 1 displays the improvement in fewer relapses and fewer dis-

Figure 1: The Effect of a New CMRC Pass Policy

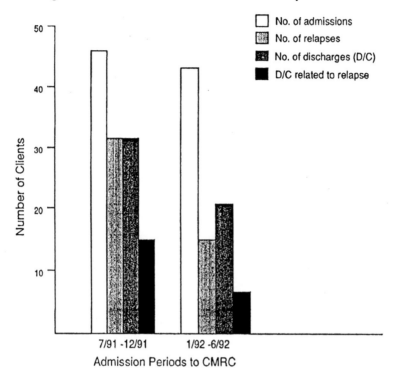

charges as a result of relapse. From the period July 1 to December 31, 1991, 47 residents were admitted to the CMRC. These 47 residents had 32 relapse events and 32 discharges; 15 (47%) of the 32 discharges were related to relapse. Of the 47 residents admitted, 15 (32%) were discharged-related-to-relapse.

The new pass policy became effective January 1, 1992. During the six months following the implementation of the new pass policy, 43 residents who were admitted subsequently had 15 relapse events and 21 discharges; seven (33%) of the 21 discharges were related to relapse. Of the 43 residents admitted during this time, seven (16%) were discharged-related-to-relapse. As demonstrated by Figure 1 the number of clients in discharges-related-to-relapse was essentially cut in half after the implementation of the new pass policy (15 to 7).

IMPLEMENTATION

The evolution of this project is marked by the support and assistance of the VA system; locally, regionally, and at the VA Central Office (VACO) level. The type and amount of support was proportionately related to the phase of project planning, activation and subsequent implementation. Support from VACO and local senior management was important from the outset. Hines VAH management provided support for the use of the building which houses the program. By good fortune, the building was available because of the construction and timely occupation of a replacement psychiatric facility. The Mental Health and Behavioral Science Department, VACO, provided funds making possible the renovation of the old psychiatric facility. Additionally, support and approval by hospital management allowed for the acquisition, storage and use of furniture and other needed equipment.

Social Work Service hospital staff entered into a contractual relationship with Northwestern University. Team building, role clarification and task assignment were vital. It was necessary to develop and enhance systems of communication between research staff, clinical research staff, clinical program staff and hospital staff in multiple departments. Senior management exemplified positive modeling and validated the active support of at least 12 other services within the hospital. Because this type program and the established grant requirements were unparalleled in VA, the infrastructure of the hospital system required some adjustments.

In the developmental phase, planning was a central focus that related to physical plant construction updates and activation, staff recruitment and training needs, role negotiation, conflict resolution, and publication plans and guidelines. Ad hoc committees were initially established to develop structure, policy and procedures for program operation and to interview key staff. Consultation with hospital administrative and other clinical services were engaged, e.g., Dietary, Personnel, Rehabilitation Medicine and Fiscal Services, to name a few. This was necessary because of modification to the hospital's infrastructure and the multidisciplinary nature of the project staff. Social Work Service in customary care is responsible administratively and professionally for the social workers in customary care. In the experimental CMRC program, in order to expedite CMRC staff hiring and program start-up, the clinical program was organizationally aligned with Research Service. Supervision of program staff remained with Social Work Service. The Co-Principal Investigator/Chief, Social Work Service supervises the customary care social work staff and CMRC program coordinator. The CMRC program coordinator, in turn, is the immediate supervisor for all experimental clinical program staff. He is assisted with consultation by the Chief, Social Work Service and two customary care social work supervisors who are also Co-Investigators of the project.

Staff education, clinical program development and research have been central in implementing the program and treating this homeless population. Clinical co-investigators have conducted seminars for research staff covering issues of street drugs, identification and management of suicidal behavior and DSM-III-R diagnoses with their behavioral manifestations. Formal and informal meetings have occurred with all levels of customary staff to clarify study protocols, randomizations and to gain access to hospital services for special needs.

Specific roles and responsibilities of personnel involved in the CMRC had to be defined. The case managers and the substance abuse counselors, as hired, were familiar with customary non-case management treatment models. In their roles as case managers, however, they functioned more as general practitioners referring residents to specialists while retaining overall responsibility for coordination of treatment, crisis intervention and monitoring.

Various processes were used to encourage communication and cooperation. Initially, clinical and research staff were competitive and had problems understanding each other's perspectives. As time progressed and after many meetings, trust was developed, experiences were shared and a sense of common ownership of the project developed. Now clinicians and researchers view themselves as a team with a positive working relationship.

Team building has been an integral component of this project. Diverse methods and techniques have been utilized to achieve team building activities and span all levels of the clinical and research staff. Full team meetings, chaired by the Principal Investigator, in the beginning stages were held weekly, and are now held monthly. This meeting is attended by all clinical and research administrative staff. The focus of the meeting is on research and clinical program updates, planning, problem identification and problem resolution.

For the CMRC staff, several types of meetings are held weekly, such as: interdisciplinary planning and review meetings, clinical consultation, daily report and shift change meetings and meetings with residents. Although purposes vary, all meetings include planning, identifying and solving problems, and addressing administrative and clinical issues.

Marketing of the project has also been important. Briefings with customary and experimental staff have been essential for achieving the planned administration of the project. Marketing was an ongoing process designed to enhance service acquisition, clarify misconceptions and maximize the involvement of hospital and community personnel.

When unique problems were encountered, special systems were developed. They were parallel to, yet different from, the usual organizational structure. The special systems included arranging for independent budget management, food purchases and other products and services needed. A designation of "residents" was given to the study participants rather than "patients" for distinction of their non-bed status and to signal transition from a sick to a healthy role.

Since the VAMC is a large campus, placement of a residential component has some different complexities than those experienced in community placements. However, in the VA's version of the "not in my backyard" syndrome, VA staff who occupy residences on the VA grounds were concerned about how the program participants would be controlled and identified from the usual patient population. Rules were developed governing areas that were off limits. Residents were also given picture ID badges.

CONCLUSION

The present project attempts a randomized field experiment testing the relative efficacy of a case management intervention for a specific subgroup of homeless, substance abusing veterans that contains a three to six month residential component. By comparing this experimental intervention to customary care, we hope to determine whether a more intensive intervention with homeless veterans has any greater efficacy than customary inpatient detoxification for patients who are non-compliant with recommendations for outpatient treatment and referral. Although the social, economic, and psychiatric complications of substance abuse disorders among the homeless veteran population provides a dramatic challenge to any experimental intervention, it is clear that existing systems for this subgroup of homeless, non-compliant, substance abusing veterans are not fully adequate to meet the needs of these individuals. The Northwestern/Hines project results should help clinicians and VA policy makers understand more about how to allocate substance abuse inpatient versus outpatient and/or residential care among a specific subgroup of non-compliant, homeless substance abuse patients that utilize the VA health care system.

REFERENCES

Castaneda, R., Lifshutz, H., & Galenter, M. (1992). Treatment compliance after detoxification among highly disadvantaged alcoholics, *American Journal of Drug and Alcohol Abuse, 18*(2), 223-234.

Goering, P., Wasylenk, D., Farkas, M., Lancee, W., & Ballantine, R. (1988). What difference does case management make? *Hospital and Community Psychiatry, 39*(3), 272-276.

Kanter, J. (1989). Clinical case management: Definition, principles, components. *Hospital and Community Psychiatry, 40*(4), 361-368.

McAdams, D. (1991). *Total Quality Management: The Strategic Imperative (T.Q.M. Training Manual for Hines VA Hospital)*. Houston: American Productivity and Quality Center.

McRae, J., Higgins, M., Lycam, C., & Sherman, W. (1990). What happens to patients after five years of intensive case management stops? *Hospital and Community Psychiatry, 41*(2), 175-179.

Moos, R.H. (1992). VA substance abuse care: What we need to know. Paper presented at annual meeting of VA Health Services Research and Development Service, Washington, D.C.

Thompson, J.P., Anderson, T.R., Boeringa, J.A. (1992). How to counsel homeless veterans. *VA Practitioner, 9*(5), p. 27-28.

Treatment for the Dually Diagnosed Homeless: Program Models and Implementation Experience: Los Angeles

Elizabeth A. McGlynn, PhD
Julie Boynton, MSW
Sally C. Morton, PhD
Brian M. Stecher, PhD
Charles Hayes, BA
Jerome V. Vaccaro, MD
M. Audrey Burnam, PhD

SUMMARY. This paper describes a research demonstration project currently underway in Los Angeles county. The study is a randomized evaluation of treatment strategies for homeless persons with serious mental and substance use disorders. This paper describes the

Drs. McGlynn, Morton, Stecher, and Burnam are affiliated with RAND; Ms. Boynton and Mr. Hayes are affiliated with Social Model Recovery Systems; and Dr. Vaccaro is affiliated with the University of California at Los Angeles, Neuropsychiatric Institute and the Veterans Administration.

Address correspondence to: Elizabeth A. McGlynn, RAND, 1700 Main Street, P.O. Box 2138, Santa Monica, CA 90407-2138.

This research was supported under a cooperative agreement from the National Institute on Alcohol Abuse and Alcoholism.

[Haworth co-indexing entry note]: "Treatment for the Dually Diagnosed Homeless: Program Models and Implementation Experience: Los Angeles." McGlynn, Elizabeth A. et al. Co-published simultaneously in the *Alcoholism Treatment Quarterly* (The Haworth Press, Inc.) Vol. 10, No. 3/4, 1993, pp. 171-186; and: *Treatment of the Chemically Dependent Homeless: Theory and Implementation in Fourteen American Projects* (ed: Kendon J. Conrad, Cheryl I. Hultman, and John S. Lyons) The Haworth Press, Inc., 1993, pp. 171-186. Multiple copies of this article/chapter may be purchased from The Haworth Document Delivery Center [1-800-3-HAWORTH: 9:00 a.m. - 5:00 p.m. (EST)].

171

study population, the treatment philosophy underlying the programs being studied, the design of the two treatment programs, and implementation experiences occurring during the first year of project operations. The existing residential program staff was able to adapt to treating a different client population. Considerable challenges were encountered in implementing the new nonresidential program. Implementation of the randomized design and longitudinal follow-up have been successful.

INTRODUCTION

Among the homeless population, about one-quarter also have both a severe mental disorder and a history of substance abuse. This "dually diagnosed" group experiences considerable difficulty in obtaining both basic services (e.g., housing, food, clothing) and treatment services for their mental disorder and substance abuse. Although a few programs have been developed in recent years to serve this population, there have been almost no efforts to systematically evaluate the effectiveness of these programs. This paper describes a research demonstration project currently underway in Los Angeles county that is designed to evaluate two treatment programs for the dually diagnosed, one residential and one nonresidential, and to compare the effectiveness of these programs with each other and with a control group. This paper will describe the target population, the philosophy of social model recovery that is reflected in the programs that are being evaluated, design of the programs, and our experiences with program and research implementation. Because the research is still underway, we will not report on preliminary outcomes of treatment.

The study population is drawn primarily from the westside area of Los Angeles county; respondents must meet three major eligibility criteria to participate in the study. First, the individual must have a history of unstable living arrangements in the six months prior to study entry. This criterion can be satisfied in a number of different ways including: (a) the person was homeless at least one night during the past month; (b) the person was homeless at least seven nights during the past six months; (c) the person lived in two or more dependent living arrangements over the past six months.[1] Second, the individual must have symptoms consistent with an Axis I mental disorder (e.g., major depression, schizophrenia). Third, the individual must

---

1. Dependent living arrangements are operationalized as institutions (e.g., hospital or jail) if the individual had nowhere else to live, had a hotel or motel room paid for with a voucher, or was staying with friends or family because the person had no other place to go.

have symptoms consistent with a substance use disorder. The Diagnostic Interview Schedule (DIS) is used to screen for the presence of substance use and mental disorders (Robins et al., 1981; Koegel and Burnam, 1992).

We elected to focus on this population for a number of reasons. First, the dually diagnosed represent a significant subgroup of the homeless population. For example, a study in California found that about one-third of the homeless had a serious mental illness and almost three-quarters of those individuals also had a substance abuse problem, suggesting that about one-quarter of all homeless persons in California may be dually diagnosed (Vernez et al., 1988). Other studies support this high prevalence of severe mental and substance use disorders among the homeless (Koegel et al., 1988; Fischer and Breakey, 1991; Drake, Osher, and Wallach, 1991). Second, the dually diagnosed have significant problems functioning in everyday life (Drake and Wallach, 1989) and they are likely to be home- less longer and incarcerated more often (Roth and Bean, 1986). Third, the current system, which tends to treat separately the problems of mental illness and substance abuse, has had difficulty providing effective treat- ments for this population (Ridgely, Osher, and Talbott, 1987; Vernez et al., 1988; Cooper, Brown, and Anglin, 1989; Ridgely, Goldman, and Willen- bring, 1990). For example, treatment outcomes in substance abuse pro- grams tend to be worse for those who also have psychiatric symptoms or diagnoses (Gillis and Keet, 1969; LaPorte et al., 1981; McLellan et al., 1983; Baekeland et al., 1973). There is a recognition among treatment providers that new models must be tried and tested and this process has just begun (Kofoed et al., 1986; Hellerstein and Meehan, 1987; Ries and Ellingson, 1989; Bond et al.,1991; Drake et al., in press). Such studies will substantially improve the ability of public sector service systems to use scarce resources to provide an appropriate mix of services.

The service demonstration program described here is being tested on the westside of Los Angeles county in a 12-square mile suburban area that contains two beach communities (Venice and Santa Monica). Los Angeles county has the second largest concentration of homeless in the country and the westside has the second largest concentration of homeless within the county, with approximately 1500 persons homeless in this area on any given night. There is little low income housing available on the westside and there are few services available that are specifically designed for this population. River Community, the residential program included in this study, is one of the few programs in the county designed specifically for the dually diagnosed population.

Some descriptive information about respondents who were enrolled in the study as of May 1992 is shown in Table 1. The respondents are

Table 1

Characteristics of Participants in Evaluation of Treatment Programs
for Persons with Dual Diagnoses (N = 88)

Characteristic	Number of Participants	Percent of Participants
Age		
19-29	15	17
30-49	67	76
50+	6	7
Gender		
Male	74	84
Female	14	16
Race		
White	49	56
Black	29	33
Hispanic	5	6
Other	5	6
Meets DIS*Criteria for:		
Major depression (lifetime)	73	83
Mania (lifetime)	40	45
Schizophrenia (lifetime)	44	50
Drug dependence (recent)	48	55
Alcohol dependence (recent)	55	63
Primary substance of abuse:		
Alcohol	41	47
Cocaine/crack	31	35
Cannabis/marijuana	9	10
Other	7	8
Age first homeless		
<15	9	10
15-18	12	14
19-29	26	30
30-39	22	25
40+	19	22
Total time client has spent homeless		
<6 months	4	5
6 months to 1 year	12	14
1-2 years	17	19
2-5 years	23	26
>5 years	32	36

* Diagnostic Interview Schedule

dominantly young, white or black males with major depression who abuse alcohol and cocaine. Almost one-fourth became homeless before they were 18; more than one-third have been homeless for five years or more.

PHILOSOPHY OF TREATMENT

The goal of social model recovery is to assist clients in developing an independent and satisfying life in the community through abstinence from alcohol and street drugs and by enhancing their social and vocational abilities. A fundamental principle is that this goal can best be achieved in small, structured, therapeutic environments in which clients learn by interaction with one another, with staff, and with the surrounding community.

Seven major principles have guided Social Model Recovery Systems, the parent organization that is responsible for River Community and Night Moves, in the development of its social model recovery programs:

- Abstinence from alcohol and all non-life sustaining drugs is a prerequisite for effective program participation.
- The program environment is an essential aspect of the treatment process. The environment must be designed and maintained in a manner that dignifies both clients and staff.
- A structured schedule of activities is essential to the creation of new patterns of behavior.
- A comprehensive therapeutic milieu with services provided by a well trained staff team is essential.
- A strong, long-term case management effort is essential. The case management component must be integrated with both residential and community outreach efforts.
- People working together can help each other to recover from mutual, shared problems. Participation in self-help groups is emphasized as an essential and ongoing aspect of recovery.
- Each client will be respected and valued as someone with an important contribution to make to the community and society as a whole.

PROGRAM DESIGN

In this section we provide a general description of the program elements, noting key differences between the residential (River Community) and nonresidential (Night Moves) programs. These elements are summarized in Table 2.

Table 2

Summary of Key Program Elements

Program Element	Description
Curriculum-Based Groups	
Thought/Mood Disorder Education	Psychoeducational groups provide a foundation for understanding mental illness from the social and medical perspectives. Clients taught to identify illness symptoms to enhance ability to seek help earlier. Information on medication side effects and skills for communicating with psychiatrists about symptoms and side effects.
Alcohol/Drug Education	Psychoeducational groups help clients explore their individual patterns of substance abuse. Physical effects of substance abuse are examined. Behavioral alternatives to substance use taught.
Stress and Coping	Clients taught how to identify life stressors. Behavior modification techniques used to improve skills for coping with stress.
Feeling Good	Clients learn to explore feelings of anger, sadness, happiness, depression, and grief within a framework of coping with these feelings without using drugs or alcohol.
Family Systems	Clients explore family issues related to dysfunction. Process of discovery and healing begun.
12 Step Meetings	Clients attend AA and NA meetings in the community to build a support group for long-term recovery. Staff help clients learn to participate in these groups.
Community Meetings	Process group designed to address issues related to living (River Community) or receiving treatment (Night Moves) in a group setting. Used to deal with problems that threaten the health, safety, or integrity of the group or treatment environment.

Table 2 (cont.)

Summary of Key Program Elements

Program Element	Description
Resident Council	Process group run by clients without staff present allows an opportunity to discuss problems within the client groups. Also used for making chore assignments and providing input to program decisions.
Individual Counseling/Case Management	Each client is assigned a primary counselor who is responsible for working with client from admission to discharge to develop individual treatment plan and monitor progress toward personal goals. At Night Moves, case management is used to help link clients to benefits and other needed services.
Medication	Most clients in this program require psychiatric medications. At River Community, medications are kept in a central, locked storage area. At Night Moves, clients are responsible for keeping track of their own medications to reinforce personal responsibility for following treatment regimens.
Personal Time	Clients are taught how to plan activities for their leisure time that do not involve drug and alcohol use.
Recreation	Organized recreational activities are designed to teach clients how to socialize in a sober environment. Sports, movies, and museum visits are done as a group.
Drug Testing	Abstinence from alcohol and drugs (other than those prescribed by a physician) is a mandatory feature of the River Community. Night Moves has a somewhat different policy–client cannot be drunk or high in order to participate in program activities. Testing is done in both programs at regular intervals and randomly. At River Community, failure to maintain abstinence is grounds for discharge.

Social Model Recovery Systems has developed educational curricula for many program groups. The five groups are described briefly in the table. The curricula are divided into weekly modules that are independent of one another because clients enter treatment throughout the course of the year (rather than in cohorts). Since the modules are independent, the client does not have to have been present at the prior session to understand material in the current session. Clients who remain for the entire treatment program (6 months) will receive all curriculum modules.

The comprehensive treatment program includes group and individual counseling as well as attendance at Alcoholics Anonymous, Narcotics Anonymous and other self-help groups. Assertive case management is a key element of the nonresidential program.

Abstinence from alcohol and other drugs is required in the residential program in order to remain in treatment. In the nonresidential program, there is somewhat more flexibility; clients are not allowed to participate in programs if they have been drinking alcohol or using drugs that day, but the staff works with clients to keep them engaged in treatment. Drug testing is used in both programs (scheduled and random) to confirm maintenance of abstinence.

Clients have daily chore assignments; participation in planning, preparing, setting up, serving and cleaning up after meals is valuable both as a means of building an independent living skill and as a vehicle for encouraging productive group activity.

The structured program has three distinct phases. Phase I emphasizes the engagement process; Phase II emphasizes addressing personal and interpersonal issues; and, Phase III emphasizes dealing with separation from treatment and placement into the community at large. A graduation ceremony is held at the conclusion of Phase III to celebrate successful program completion.

The program orientation recognizes that people do not make progress toward recovery at the same rate. The phases are designed to make allowances for individual differences. The criteria for advancement from one phase to the next is based on completion and/or progress toward goals and objectives as outlined in individual treatment/goal plans. In light of this, some clients are able to graduate more quickly than others.

PROGRAM IMPLEMENTATION

The purpose of this project was to replicate a residential treatment program for individuals with major mental disorder and substance use disorder in a nonresidential setting and to evaluate the effectiveness of these two programs as compared to each other and to a control group. The residential treatment program, River Community, has been in operation in Los Angeles county since 1987. Through the research demonstration project, River Community began offering a new service link; homeless persons from the westside were eligible to be admitted directly through the project without having to spend three to four months on the County's waiting list. The nonresidential program was created by the project and provided services not previously available in the county. Thus, the implementation issues for the two programs were quite different and will be discussed separately.

River Community: Issues for an Established Program

River Community staff had two sets of concerns about the effect of this research project on their program. First, they were concerned about the potential intrusiveness of the research on program operations. Second, they were concerned about the influx of a homeless population on the social model recovery environment. In general, staff concerns in both of these areas have not materialized to any great degree.

Staff was concerned about the intention to randomly assign clients to treatment. Currently, clients entering through the usual county referral process spend about 4 months on a waiting list. To maintain their place in the queue, clients must keep in regular contact with the intake coordinator. The belief was that such clients arrive at the program with fairly strong motivations to succeed in treatment. Would random assignment with immediate access result in clients with lower motivation? The final answer to this question awaits the analysis of the full data set, but a preliminary indication is that study clients are behaving similarly to non-study clients in terms of length-of-stay and patterns-of-stay; roughly the same proportion of study clients and non-study clients complete the program. Both study and non-study clients who stay in the program at least one month are likely to complete treatment.

In order to reduce the sources of variation between the residential and nonresidential programs, we required that the same curriculum be used at both programs and that it be run on the same time schedule. We also revised the curriculum prior to beginning the study. River Community staff were concerned that they might lose some flexibility in running their groups. In the beginning, there were some problems with implementing the new curriculum. Staff were overly concerned with following the precise content outline and ended up lecturing and reading more material than had been the case prior to the research. Clients complained about the way the curriculum was being delivered and the deputy director worked with staff on achieving a balance between following the intent of the curriculum and adapting the presentation to their own particular style. As staff became more comfortable with the new curriculum, their group facilitation styles also began to re-emerge.

There was a variety of concerns related to introducing large numbers of homeless individuals into the program. There are 32 beds at River Community and 10 of them are designated study beds; prior to the study, only a handful of homeless clients had been admitted. Staff concerns revolved around clients making the transition from street behavior to behavior appropriate in a structured program, hygiene and health issues, and whether study clients would have lower functional levels, be psychiatrically unstable, and be able to detoxify safely in the social model setting. There have been somewhat greater challenges breaking through the street behaviors clients bring into the program. In particular, the therapeutic groups challenge clients to share information about themselves that would not normally be an acceptable part of street behavior. Study clients may take somewhat longer to participate fully in the groups, but fewer problems have been encountered than were anticipated. The greatest health and hygiene issue has been that study clients often arrive at the program without appropriate clothing. A clothing drive was held at RAND early in the study to provide an inventory of clothes from which to draw. Subsequently, River Community has worked to develop other sources of clothing for these clients. Although many study clients function at lower cognitive levels than non-study clients, this has not presented any serious problem in the educational or process groups. Many of the study clients are not stabilized on medications when they arrive at the program and the psychiatrist has been more actively involved in assessments and prescribing medications than is typical for non-study clients. Detoxification has not presented the problems feared because this population detoxifies "naturally" monthly when they run out of resources to purchase alcohol or drugs. Where necessary, arrangements have been made for medical detoxification prior to program entry.

Night Moves: Replicating an Existing Model in a New Setting

Replicating successful programs always presents an implementation challenge; when replication requires modification, such as shifting from a residential to a nonresidential setting, the challenge increases. Many of the implementation problems encountered in this demonstration revolved around the key differences in operating residential and nonresidential programs. We will discuss five implementation issues: developing operating policies and procedures, designing the curriculum, staffing/personnel, developing a program culture, and start-up time requirements.

Developing Operating Policies and Procedures. The most difficult challenge faced in developing policies for the nonresidential program was designing an abstinence policy that recognized clients living on the street would have difficulty getting and maintaining sobriety while challenging clients to make progress toward continuous abstinence. After trying fairly rigid standards (e.g., three episodes of non-abstinence) with program termination as a consequence, Night Moves has evolved toward a policy of setting individual goals and behavior contracts. In general, more allowances are made for clients who are just beginning the program and increased expectations are placed on those who are further along.

A related challenge that is unique to the nonresidential setting is setting a required level of program attendance. Originally, the program operated seven days per week and clients were required to attend every day. Failure to show up at the program, without staff permission, three days in a row was grounds for discharge from the program. Currently the program is open five days per week and clients are expected to attend each evening. However, staff works with clients to establish attendance policies that meet individual needs. In the beginning, nightly attendance may be difficult for a client to achieve; later on, some clients acquire jobs or are engaged in other recovery-related activities that represent positive transitions to long-term recovery in the community. Night Moves staff maintains a flexible approach to individual needs.

Program Curriculum. As discussed above, the curriculum groups were designed to be identical in content across the two programs. However, some differences in approach were required for the nonresidential program. Clients in the two programs face somewhat different situations in their day-to-day lives which meant developing some different examples for role plays, illustrations of key concepts, and suggestions for practicing some of the behavior modification techniques presented during the educational modules.

A more significant problem in the early stages of the program was that the new staff had not ever presented educational modules in a treatment setting. We did not allot sufficient time for training new staff on the use of modules and the program director was not effective in setting aside time for staff to prepare for the modules. As a result, the modules were often just read to clients–hardly an engaging technique. More recently, efforts have been made to provide staff with training and preparation time.

Staffing/Personnel. In developing a new program, particularly one that presents as many challenges as the nonresidential program, it is essential to hire a highly trained and flexible staff. One of the difficulties for dual diagnosis treatment programs is that there are no training programs that are producing individuals who are specifically trained to treat this population. So, one must hire staff who are trained in either substance abuse treatment or mental health treatment. It is important to hire staff, however, who are capable of being flexible with respect to the treatment principles learned in their primary training area. One of the hallmarks of dual diagnosis treatment is the need to blend the principles of substance abuse and mental health treatment. In particular, considerations of when to confront clients in order to break down denial systems versus taking a nonconfrontational stance with the client require careful clinical judgment. Night Moves had a complete turnover in staff in the first nine months of operation. What was learned from that experience guided the subsequent round of hiring, resulting in a staff better suited to the program requirements.

Case management skills were particularly important for the nonresidential program. Considerable attention has been devoted to training staff in the principles of assertive case management. More staff time at Night Moves is devoted to the variety of case management activities because clients in this program require attention to assist them in meeting basic living needs.

Developing a Program Culture. The essence of social model programs is their philosophic approach to clients and to the process of treatment. Developing a team approach to treatment is one of the essential elements. A distinguishing feature of social model programs is that clients are considered part of the team along with staff. Although each group has specific roles, there is a recognition that both contribute to the treatment process. This is difficult for staff trained in more medically-oriented delivery systems to adopt. One of the ways Night Moves attempted to promote this attitude was through the structure of the facility. The staff have desks in the front room, but not individual offices, and entry to the program is through the staff area. This encourages the mingling of staff and clients and enhances the sense of teamwork among the staff. However, based on some of our process evaluation and ethnographic work, it appears that the culture at Night Moves is quite different from that at River Community. Night Moves is more staff-directed and has more of a medical model orientation than River Community.

Start-Up Time Requirements. Due to time pressures related to the length of the grant, we allotted just three months to pilot the new nonresidential treatment program. Clearly, that was not enough time to develop a stable, functioning program. Although it would be difficult to achieve within the context of research, a one-year start-up is probably more reasonable. In discussing some of the implementation problems we encountered in Night Moves start-up with staff from River Community, we discovered considerable similarities. In its initial year of operation, River Community underwent considerable staff turnover and changes in the structure of key program elements. We had, of course, hoped to short circuit the learning curve by building on the experiences of River Community, but the design of a nonresidential program and some of the organizational conflicts encountered at the beginning of the project offset the benefits of some of our learning. In retrospect, while new programs can always learn implementation lessons from existing programs, in all likelihood they will encounter new problems that will take some time to resolve. To make fair comparisons in evaluating programs, researchers should allow time for a program to stabilize before studying performance (particularly if comparisons are being made to an established program).

RESEARCH IMPLEMENTATION

Conducting randomized evaluations of treatment programs for persons with dual diagnoses presented a challenge for the research staff as well. Careful screening, training, and monitoring of field staff is essential to maintaining the quality and integrity of the research design. The data collection process begins with a brief (10 minute) screener to determine whether the individual meets the criteria for homelessness, presence of a mental disorder, and presence of a substance abuse problem. Respondents are given two dollars for completing the screener. Those who "pass" the screener are asked to take a longer (1 hour) diagnostic interview to confirm the presence of mental and substance use disorders. We have had excellent response rates at both of these stages. As of October 1992, 92 percent of those approached (n = 969) agreed to take the screener and 88 percent of those eligible to take the diagnostic interview (n = 557) agreed to do so. Respondents are given ten dollars for completing the diagnostic interview.

Individuals who meet the eligibility criteria for study participation are then given two weeks to consider whether or not they wish to enroll. This delay is at odds with standard practice in the substance abuse recovery field where individuals are immediately placed into a treatment program after an "intervention" has taken place. However, our experience in the pilot study was that while almost everyone agreed to participate in the study, only about one-half ever showed up. Our concern was that clients were not making an informed, non-coerced decision to participate; because of the rapport they had built with the interviewer during the diagnostic interview it might be easier to agree to participate to please the interviewer than to refuse.

From a research perspective, we also wanted to include in the study only those who really intended to accept their program assignment (residential, nonresidential, or control). Consistent with what we found during the pilot study, and using this two week "cooling off" period, 63 percent of those who were eligible to participate (n = 416) agreed to enroll. Among those refusing to enroll, about half never returned (passive refusal) and the other half told the interviewer they were not going to enroll. The process of random assignment worked quite well; no problems were encountered in the field.

We also obtain data from study participants at 3, 6, and 9 months after enrollment. Respondents are given ten dollars for each of these follow-up interviews. To enhance our ability to locate clients for these interviews we obtain a substantial amount of information from clients at enrollment about where they hang out, where they pick up benefits checks, and what friends or family members generally know where they can be found. In addition, respondents who get in touch with research staff to schedule follow-up interview appointments are given an extra dollar. As much as possible, interviewers follow the same respondents throughout the research process and are encouraged to locate as many respondents as possible. Thus far, our response rates are at 87 percent for the 3-month, 83 percent for the 6-month, and 76 percent for the 9-month interview. Some of the lower response for the 9-month is accounted for by individuals we have located (89 percent) but are unable to interview (e.g., because they are in a jail that is located too far away and without a non-monitored phone line).

CONCLUSION

We have presented an overview of the target population we are studying along with a description of the treatment philosophy, program design, and program and research implementation issues. It is premature to speculate on the success of either of these programs in treating persons with serious mental illness and substance abuse, but considerable progress has been made in developing and implementing a nonresidential treatment model for this population; we are encouraged about its potential contribution to the service delivery system in our community. We have also demonstrated that it is possible to use rigorous research methods and longitudinal designs in evaluating the effectiveness of treatment for the homeless who are dually diagnosed.

REFERENCES

Baekeland, F., Lundwall, L., Shanahan, T.J. (1973). Correlates of patient attrition in the outpatient treatment of alcoholism. *J Nerv Ment Dis,* 157, 99-107.

Bond, G.R., McDonel, E.C., Miller, E.P., Pensec, M. (1991). Assertive community treatment and reference groups: An evaluation of their effectiveness for young adults with serious mental illness and substance abuse problems. *Psychosocial Rehab J,* 15, 31-43.

Cooper, L., Brown, V.B., Anglin, M.D. (1989). Multiple diagnosis: Aspects and issues in substance abuse. Unpublished paper for the State of California, Alcohol and Drug Program.

Drake, R.E., McHugo, G., Noordsy, D.L. (in press). A pilot study of outpatient treatment of alcoholism in schizophrenia: Four-year outcomes. *Am J Psych.*

Drake, R.E., Osher, F.C., and Wallach, M.A. (1991). Homelessness and dual diagnosis. *Amer Psych,* 46, 1149-1158.

Drake, R.E., Wallach, M.A. (1989). Substance abuse among the chronic mentally ill. *Hosp and Comm Psych,* 40, 10.

Fischer, P.J., and Breakey, W.R. (1991). The epidemiology of alcohol, drug, and mental disorders among homeless persons. *Amer Psych,* 46(11).

Gillis, L.S., Keet, M. (1969). Prognostic factors and treatment results in hospitalized alcoholics. *Q J Stud Alcohol,* 30, 426-427.

Hellerstein, D.J., Meehan, B. (1987). Outpatient group therapy for schizophrenic substance abusers. *Amer J Psych,* 144(10), 1337-1339.

Koegel, P., and Burnam, M.A. (1992). Issues in the assessment of mental disorders among the homeless: An empirical approach. In Robertson, M.J., and Greenblatt, M. (eds.), *Homelessness: The National Perspective,* New York: Plenum Press.

Koegel, P. et al. (1988). The prevalence of specific psychiatric disorders among homeless individuals in the inner-city of Los Angeles. *Arch Gen Psych,* 45, 1085-1092.

Kofoed, L., Kania, J., Walsh, T., Atkinson, R.M. (1986). Outpatient treatment of patients with substance abuse and coexisting psychiatric disorders. *Amer J Psych,* 143, 7.

LaPorte, D.J., McClellan, A.T., O'Brien, C.P., Marshall, J.R. (1981). Treatment response in psychiatrically impaired drug abusers. *Compr Psychiatry,* 22, 411-419.

McLellan, A.T., Luborsky, L., Woody, G.E., O'Brien, C.P., Marshall, J.R. (1983). Predicting response to alcohol and drug abuse treatment: Role of psychiatric severity. *Arch Gen Psychiatry,* 40, 620-625.

Ridgely, M.S., Goldman, H.H., Willenbring, M. (1990). Barriers to the care of persons with dual diagnoses: Organizational and financing issues. *Schizophrenia Bulletin,* 16(1), 123-132.

Ridgely, M.S., Osher, F.C., Talbott, J.A. (1987). Chronic mentally ill young adults with substance abuse problems: Treatment and training issues. Unpublished paper for the University of Maryland School of Medicine.

Ries, R.K., and Ellingson, T. (1981). A pilot assessment at one month of 17 dual diagnosis patients. *Hosp and Comm Psych*, 41, 1230-1233.

Roth, D., Bean, G.J., Jr. (1986). New perspectives on homelessness: Findings from a statewide epidemiological study. *Hosp and Comm Psych*, 37, 712-719.

Vernez, G., Burnam, M.A., McGlynn, E.A., Trude, S., Mittman, B.S. (1988). *Review of California's Program for the Homeless Mentally Disabled*, The RAND Corporation, Publication No. R-3631-CDMH.

CASE MANAGEMENT: DENVER

Intensive Case Management for Homeless People with Alcohol and Other Drug Problems: Denver

Michael W. Kirby, Jr., PhD
G. Nicholas Braucht, PhD

SUMMARY. An intensive case management program designed to be effective with homeless persons affected by alcohol and other drug prob-

Michael W. Kirby, Jr. is Executive Director, Arapahoe House Comprehensive Substance Abuse Center, 8801 Lipan Street, Thornton, CO 80221. G. Nicholas Braucht is Professor of Psychology, Department of Psychology, University of Denver, Denver, CO 80208.

The preparation of this chapter was supported by Cooperative Agreement Grant No. 5U01AA08778 to the University of Denver from the Homeless Demonstration and Evaluation Branch of the National Institute on Alcohol Abuse and Alcoholism.

[Haworth co-indexing entry note]: "Intensive Case Management for Homeless People with Alcohol and Other Drug Problems: Denver." Kirby, Michael W., Jr., and G. Nicholas Braucht. Co-published simultaneously in the *Alcoholism Treatment Quarterly* (The Haworth Press, Inc.) Vol. 10, No. 3/4, 1993, pp. 187-200; and: *Treatment of the Chemically Dependent Homeless: Theory and Implementation in Fourteen American Projects* (ed: Kendon J. Conrad, Cheryl I. Hultman, and John S. Lyons) The Haworth Press, Inc., 1993, pp. 187-200. Multiple copies of this article/chapter may be purchased from The Haworth Document Delivery Center [1-800-3-HAWORTH: 9:00 a.m. - 5:00 p.m. (EST)].

lems was implemented and rigorously evaluated. The service demonstration site for the Denver project was Arapahoe House, Colorado's largest and most comprehensive substance abuse treatment center. The evaluation research efforts were conducted by the University of Denver. This project implemented an innovative model of case management, in which case managers operated in dyads and with a small caseload of clients. This model was conceived as an optimal strategy to bind clients to the continuum of substance abuse services within Arapahoe House and to link clients to other needed services and benefits in the community.

INTRODUCTION

The Denver homeless demonstration project has been designed to implement and rigorously evaluate a new model of intensive case management. This model takes the form of pairs or *dyads* of case managers who work with the target population of homeless persons affected by alcohol and other drugs. Within this model, each case manager dyad shares a low caseload–never to exceed 17 clients per dyad–and frequency and consistency of client contacts are emphasized.

The intensive case management (ICM) program described in this chapter was implemented in an existing comprehensive substance abuse services agency known as Arapahoe House. As an overlay to this existing continuum of services, the dyadic ICM program has been intended to forge linkages for each individual client to the services that are most appropriate to his or her needs. Because all clients have been enrolled in either residential or outpatient treatment with Arapahoe House, case managers do not act as the primary counselors, but rather assist the clients in connecting to those agencies and services in the community that can serve as supports beyond the client's time in treatment.

We believe this model of case management offers a number of distinctive advantages over the individual case management model. The six major advantages of working in dyads are:

1. Continuity of care is enhanced for each client, even in the face of case manager absence for vacation or illness and/or even when turnover in case managers occurs;
2. Each case manager is afforded a partner who can proffer a different perspective about the client;
3. Stress is reduced, as is the overwhelming sense of responsibility frequently experienced by case managers who operate solo;
4. The strengths of two people can be combined, blending the combined experience and skills of each into an integrated whole;

5. Communication among all team members is improved; and
6. A more efficient and effective supervisory structure is possible.

A major potential disadvantage of this model lies in its cost; however, if the dyadic model is more effective in securing for clients the most appropriate individualized mix of services, this form of intensive case management may prove to be more cost-effective in the final analysis.

The evaluation of this demonstration project is an experimental one in which clients have been randomly assigned to either the intensive case management (ICM) group or to a control group that receives the "usual" care without case management. Both groups have had access to the continuum of services available through Arapahoe House. Extensive service-oriented data were collected daily. Outcome data have been taken at three points: (1) at admission into the study; (2) four months post-admission; and (3) ten months post-admission.

BACKGROUND

Setting

The Denver, Colorado Metropolitan Area. The setting for this project is the five county area which comprises metropolitan Denver. The general population contained in this area is estimated to approach 2,000,000 persons, which is a majority of the state's total population. In comparison with other urban areas, the U.S. Department of Commerce ranks this area as 90th among 336 metropolitan areas in percentage increase in growth from 1980 to 1990. Despite this growth, this decade generally was one of economic stagnation in Colorado.

Although homelessness occurs in other areas of the state, it is principally concentrated in the city and county of Denver, spreading in a trickle from the city to the other surrounding municipalities, most especially to Aurora, which is the third largest city in Colorado and contiguous to Denver.

Arapahoe House: A Comprehensive Substance Abuse Services Agency. The service demonstration site for this project is Arapahoe House, a comprehensive alcohol and drug services agency encompassing fifteen locations across the Denver metro area. Arapahoe House was established as a non-profit corporation in 1976, serving primarily Arapahoe County with detoxification and halfway house services.

In the intervening years the agency has implemented a number of additional programs and has expanded to become the largest provider of substance abuse services in Colorado. Today the primary service area for Arapahoe House is Denver and the four counties immediately surrounding it; however, the agency's residential programs serve citizens from across the state.

Arapahoe House offers a full continuum of prevention, intervention and treatment services: (a) A 32-bed non-medical detoxification program serving primarily the southern sector of Denver County, Arapahoe and Douglas Counties; (b) a 50-bed non-medical detoxification program serving the western sector of Denver and all of Jefferson County; (c) a 64-bed short-term intensive residential treatment program with a statewide service area; (d) a 10-bed intermediate treatment program, with a regional service area; (e) an 18-bed adolescent male program serving the entire state; (f) a 22-bed transitional housing program for homeless clients who have completed an intensive treatment program; (g) seven outpatient clinics strategically located in six different municipalities within the greater Denver metro area; and (h) an array of school-based programs, including high school, middle school, and elementary school services located on site in 10 Denver schools.

Research Team: The University of Denver. Responsibility for the evaluation component of the Denver homeless demonstration project was located within an evaluation research team in the Department of Psychology at the University of Denver. The research design for this project was experimental; clients who met the admission criteria were randomly assigned on a 1:1 ratio, by means of a computer-based procedure (see Braucht and Reichardt, in press), to one of two treatment conditions: (1) a continuum of substance abuse treatment services *with* intensive case management; or (2) a "usual care" comparison condition in which there was a continuum of substance abuse services with no case management. Arapahoe House provided the core continuum of substance abuse services for both groups, as well as the intensive case management program.

The research design is a longitudinal one, in which trained interviewers on the University of Denver staff are responsible for the collection of data from study clients at three major points: (1) at admission to the project; (2) four months following admission; and (3) six months following this second data collection point, which is ten months from admission.

In addition, extensive service-oriented data have been gathered on a daily basis via the agency's computerized management information system (MIS) and on a monthly basis by the University research team. The service data from both the MIS and the monthly service logs are captured to reflect the NIAAA taxonomy of services, which was designed and implemented across the participating sites in order to ensure comparable data on services. These systems yield measures in the form of units of services delivered to study clients in hour and quarter-hour units for contact-oriented services, and in units of days for residential services. The Arapahoe House MIS utilizes, as its source document, a comprehensive service log completed daily by each staff member in a service-provider role, while the data from the monthly service logs are compiled by information taken directly from study clients. This system thus assesses at a micro level the services received by each client, including all substance abuse and case management services provided by Arapahoe House, as well as services delivered by agencies external to the agency. These data will enable us to isolate specifically the elements in the treatment or case management programs that are differentially effective with this client population. (See Finney and Moos, 1989; Graham and Birchmore-Timney, 1989, for a discussion of this important issue.)

Intensive Case Management Model. Arapahoe House derives approximately 50% of its funding from contracts with various state agencies, primarily the Alcohol and Drug Abuse Division (ADAD) of the Colorado Department of Health. At the time this project was conceived and implemented, case management was not an ADAD reimbursable activity. We felt there was a pressing need, however, for a case management team that could impact appropriate clients in at least two broad ways: (1) First, within the Arapahoe House continuum of services, each discrete program sometimes tends to be disconnected from other programs. These discontinuities can lead to fragmentation and inefficiency in the delivery of services, which is especially problematic with those clients, including homeless persons, for whom continuity is essential if they are to benefit from treatment. Case management was envisioned as a service that could ensure continuity by binding these clients to programs within and across the continuum. (2) Second, case management also was viewed as the optimal strategy for effectively linking clients to services delivered by programs outside of Arapahoe House. Through an intensive case management program, we assumed that the individual service needs of clients could be addressed effectively by securing the optimal mix of services for each individual, regardless of the location of these services in the community.

Having identified the desirability of implementing a case management model, we began to consult with other service providers, primarily case managers working in community mental health centers, to plan our case management approach.

Given that all clients who are designated as appropriate for case management services are enrolled participants in one of the Arapahoe House treatment programs, we decided our case management team would primarily act as brokers and consultants while the clients are in treatment; provision of direct clinical treatment services was to remain the primary responsibility of the counselor assigned to each client.

Thus, while a client is enrolled in treatment, the case managers are relatively peripheral until the program discharge planning process is underway. The case managers assume a much more central and active role when clients are making the transition between programs. For example, as a client begins to prepare to make the transition between residential and outpatient treatment, the case managers coordinate the process and assure that stable housing is in place prior to the transfer.

This kind of case management has been characterized as "linkage" or "brokerage" in nature, as opposed to clinical or "integrated" case management, in which the case managers are directly responsible for providing traditional treatment services as well as acting as broker for other services (Harris and Bachrach, 1988; Kline et al., 1991).

The Arapahoe House dyadic model is designed to operate intensively within a maximum period of four months duration. The overarching aim of this model is to assure that each client receives the optimal blend of substance abuse and other services that are instrumental to a more independent, productive life. It is expected that the linkages and connections achieved with the client during this period will continue to serve as salient supports for the client following discharge from Arapahoe House.

The distinction frequently made between linkage versus direct service models of case management is an important and germane one for substance abuse programs that may be interested in adding a case management component. Either the case management is, in effect, an alternative services delivery system for certain targeted clients, or it must overlay the existing array of treatment services. In this project, for a variety of reasons, we decided to implement the latter model. However, experience has demonstrated to us that this distinction can be overstated. It is quite clear that, even with our model, a considerable amount of direct services are provided by case managers.

Population

Admission Criteria. The population eligible for admission into the Denver project consisted of adult homeless men and women who met all of the following six criteria: (a) Homeless according to the NIAAA criteria; (b) assessed as having an alcohol or other drug problem warranting treatment; (c) eighteen years or older; (d) no identified medical or psychiatric problems of a magnitude that would prevent active participation in this project; (e) a willingness to participate in the project; and (f) no affirmative plans to leave the Denver metropolitan area in the next twelve months.

Client Characteristics. Table I displays selected demographic characteristics for the 163 clients enrolled in the experimental group and the 160

Table I

Gender, Ethnicity, and Age Characteristics of the Intensive Case Management Group (ICM) and the Usual Care Control Group (UCG)

	Number		Percent	
	ICM	UCG	ICM	UCG
Gender				
Male	140	133	85.9	83.1
Female	23	27	14.1	16.9
Ethnicity				
White	90	92	55.2	57.5
African American	50	44	30.7	27.5
Hispanic	15	15	9.2	9.4
Other	8	9	4.9	5.6
Age at Enrollment				
18 – 19	2	0	1.3	0.0
20 – 29	43	43	26.4	26.9
30 – 39	71	70	43.6	43.8
40 – 49	40	40	24.5	25.0
50 – 59	4	6	2.5	3.8
60 – 70	3	1	1.8	0.6
Total Group	163	160	100.0	100.0

clients in the usual care comparison group. As can be seen, the groups were closely matched in terms of gender, ethnicity and age. The great majority of clients in both groups were male, with slightly less than half being members of ethnic minority groups. The most prevalent ethnic minority in this study was African American, with about 29% of the total sample. The age range was wide, but the preponderance of clients were between 20 and 50 years old at the time of enrollment.

OBJECTIVES

Outcome Objectives

The basic goal for the project was to demonstrate and evaluate the dyadic case management model, implemented in a system in which a comprehensive array of substance abuse services already exists and is generally accessible to most clients.

As stated above, outcome measures were taken at: (1) four months following enrollment; and (2) six months later, or ten months following enrollment. The outcome assessment focused on the five principal dimensions: (1) The use of alcohol and other drugs; (2) residential stability; (3) physical and mental health; (4) employment and educational attainment; and (5) overall quality of life.

Intensive Case Management Objectives

The major thesis being tested in this demonstration project is that the ICM group will demonstrate significantly higher levels of improvement in each of these five areas in comparison with the non-ICM group. More specifically, it was hypothesized that:

1. Client participants in the Intensive Case Management (ICM) group will receive more treatment and other needed services than the non-ICM control group.
2. Services received by clients in the ICM group will be more closely tailored to their individual service needs than will the services received by non-ICM clients.
3. ICM group participants will have fewer service discontinuities and fewer relapses than control group participants.
4. As a result, clients in the ICM group will show greater improvement than clients in the non-ICM control group in the five outcome domains, that is: (a) less use of alcohol and other drugs; (b) a higher degree of residential stability; (c) more improved mental and physical health; (d) higher employment and educational attainment; and (e) greater improvement in overall quality of life.

THEORY OF TREATMENT

Agency Philosophy

Clients Are Heterogeneous. Arapahoe House operates from a philosophy that explicitly recognizes that clients who present for substance abuse treatment are a heterogeneous population, and, accordingly, endeavors to match a specific mix of services to the individual constellation of needs evidenced by each person. Prospective clients are interviewed by a member of the agency's Central Assessment and Referral team, which represents the single point of entry for the agency. This team is responsible for initial screening, problem-level assessment and a recommendation for placement within the agency's continuum of services or for appropriate referral outside of the agency.

At the time clients were enrolled in the project, individual service plans were developed. These individual service plans were based upon independent estimates (by the client, by the Central Assessment and Referral Team, and by the client's initial primary service provider) of the optimal mix of services required to meet the client's service needs during the ensuing four-month treatment episode. These individual service plans were detailed plans of specific types and amounts of services, framed within the taxonomy of 49 specific types of services designed and developed by the National Institute on Alcohol Abuse and Alcoholism (1991) to cover a wide range of distinct types of services relevant to substance abusers in general and homeless substance abusers in particular. In keeping with our philosophy, the dyadic case management model is designed to provide the optimal mix of services for each client, as represented by these individual service plans. This kind of treatment matching strategy is associated with positive outcome (see Miller and Hester, 1986), and is, from our perspective, essential to the delivery of cost-effective services.

Homeless Clients Need to Be Housed First. In comparison with other clients, homeless clients generally have a more pronounced set of service needs that frequently indicate the need for a different sequence of services (Breakey, 1987). Our operating assumption is that first priority for homeless clients is *housing;* that it is fundamental that every person requires a safe, stable setting in which to reside before other needs can be effectively addressed (Wittman, 1987). Accordingly, once a client meets the criteria for admission into the Denver Homeless Project, s/he remains in an Arapahoe House residential treatment program for at least the first 30 days following admission.

Homeless Clients Need Services Located in Multiple Systems. As is clearly evident throughout the literature on this subject, homeless persons have multiple problems and needs, including housing, medical and dental care, mental health services, substance abuse services, vocational services, and benefits acquisition. In most cases, this constellation of multiple service needs cannot be adequately addressed by a single agency. Services tend to be fragmented and to be located in different systems and agencies.

Case management offers a strategy that is explicitly designed to identify the individual service needs of each client, and to match these needs with the most appropriate agency or service, regardless of location. Unfortunately, well-designed case management models frequently are undermined by the realities of inadequate resources, as well as through deficiencies in implementation.

We believe it is essential that case management be intensive. We expect that that intensity will derive from low caseloads and from the consequent opportunity (and expectation) for frequent and consistent contact between case manager and client. In the Arapahoe House dyadic Intensive Case Management model, caseloads have been designed not to exceed 17 clients per dyad. In addition, through our management information system, the frequency and duration of contacts are monitored regularly to ensure that all clients on each caseload are receiving the level of services required by this model.

Homeless Clients Need Continuity of Care. One of the foundations of case management is that it ostensibly affords continuity of care for clients. Continuity, in this context, refers to consistency of services over time, and implies that changes in the nature or level of services will be planned in advance and coordinated to ensure minimal disruption to the person who is the recipient of services.

Intensive Case Management Is Vital in Linking Clients to These Different Services. Increasingly, substance abuse programs endorse case management. An analysis of the actual practices of these programs, however, frequently reveals that the case manager has simply taken the place of the more traditional referral counselor. The primary responsibility for referral counselors is, not surprisingly, to make referrals. While it is important to refer, the referral process per se is not coterminous with case management. In our model, case management entails the forging of linkages with a network of agencies and services providers; further, once the linkages are made, the case manager monitors the quality and efficacy of these linkages and, where necessary, intervenes on the client's behalf.

Initial Interventions

There were two levels of interventions in the present project: (1) first, initial interventions were designed specifically to enhance the outreach to and engagement with homeless people who may not be frequent users of one of the area detoxification programs; (2) second, extended interventions were effected to augment the existing traditional continuum of substance abuse treatment services available from Arapahoe House.

M.O.R.E. Team. The goal was to admit to the project a mix of homeless people that was reasonably representative of the larger homeless population in Denver. Consequently, the Mobile Outreach Response Effort was created. Known locally as the M.O.R.E. team, a rotating shift of counselors operated out of our Arapahoe County detoxification program in a telephone-equipped van. While the preliminary plan called for limited hours of operation, the M.O.R.E. team was expanded to be available seven days a week, 24 hours a day. The team adhered to a regular schedule to homeless shelters, emergency rooms, and certain key locations where homeless people congregate, and also has been on call at all hours.

Homeless Stabilization Phase. In an effort to minimize client attrition due to limited residential program capacity, Arapahoe House created an additional treatment track following the normal detoxification regimen; this "homeless stabilization phase" typically spanned 2 to 5 additional days.

Extended Intervention: Dyadic Case Management Model

The extended intervention implemented in this project was *intensive case management (ICM)*. The Arapahoe House ICM model was designed for case managers to function in pairs or dyads. Each dyad of case managers works with all clients on its shared caseload. Each client thus has a relationship with a primary and a secondary case manager. As stated earlier, this model of case management derives its intensity from low caseloads, which do not exceed 17 clients per dyad, and from the expected high frequency and consistency of contact with clients. This is designed to be a proactive and assertive model of case management, that cuts across systems and agency barriers to obtain and link each client to the services and benefits that best meet his or her needs.

HISTORY OF PROJECT IMPLEMENTATION

Hiring and Training of Case Management Team

The six-person case management team was recruited from a variety of sources, including mental health, social work, social services, and from within the agency. We did not consider degrees to be of importance, and, indeed, did not particularly emphasize a background with case management. Rather, our screening and hiring process emphasized two attributes: the individual's understanding of and commitment to working with this client population in the community (not in offices), and his/her skills and experience. We sought to represent across the team the requisite areas of expertise for this project and this target population, including housing, benefits acquisition, health care, and vocational training. In addition, we endeavored to identify people with personal strength and integrity who could withstand the rigorous and sometimes overly demanding pressures that are an integral part of the case manager job. Training for the team was conducted by the Case Manager Coordinator, utilizing a set of materials she developed in concert with consultants. A training manual is available from the Case Manager Coordinator with Arapahoe House upon request.

Problem Areas and Resolution

The project represents a substantial effort in several important respects: first, it required development and refinement of a new intensive case management program, based on a dyadic model, for which there was no precedent, in a compressed period of time. Second, this model had to be implemented in a system of treatment which was well-established. Third, while the Arapahoe House staff was accustomed to research and program evaluation as ongoing activities, this project elevated these activities to a much more prominent and demanding level than had previously been the case.

The following is a summary of some of the more significant problems that emerged over the first 25 months of this project.

Continuous Residential Stability. Initially, bed dates in one of the Arapahoe House residential programs were assigned without any special priority placed on project clients. This policy produced an undesirable rate of attrition between the homeless stabilization phase in detoxification and admission into a residential program. The problem was resolved by reserving beds for project clients with immediate access following the homeless stabilization phase.

Mobile Outreach Response Effort (MORE) Team. We failed to adequately anticipate the difficulties attendant to recruiting, hiring and maintaining staff for the MORE team. This problem gradually resolved itself, through refinement in hiring practices and in improved management of the program.

Implementation of Case Management. As expected, problems were encountered in the effort to integrate the new case management team into the existing Arapahoe House continuum. These problems were resolved early in the project, primarily through a series of staff meetings designated specifically to address this problem.

Development of Resource Network and Directory. Establishing a comprehensive community resource network and directory proved to be much more difficult than we had anticipated. Although there are a multiplicity of resources for homeless people in the metro Denver area, there was no established resource network among providers, nor was there a current resources manual or directory that encompassed the available network. We have developed and published this directory and the feedback to date from providers has been uniformly positive.

Assessment of Client Motivation. Our admission criteria had to be refined, especially in the area of assessment of client motivation. In the pilot phase, some clients lied about their motivation and/or their homeless status to gain admission, principally to obtain the participant reimbursement. This problem was easily resolved by altering the method by which participant reimbursement payments were made, requiring that both the admission and discharge interviews be completed before payment was rendered.

Areas of Major Accomplishment

Coordination of Research and Treatment. Given the size and scope of this project, the relationship between the research staff at the University of Denver and the program staff at Arapahoe House has been exemplary. Communication has been excellent; staff turnover for both staffs has been non-existent; and a consistent level of mutual respect and commitment to the objectives of the project has been in evidence from the outset.

Perceived Efficacy of Dyadic Model. From a subjective programmatic perspective, the dyadic case manager model has been proven to be more efficacious than we had envisioned in the best case scenario. The three dyads work well together and clients have been the beneficiaries. There has been no turnover to date in the six case manager or Case Manager Coordinator positions.

Impact of the Project on Colorado. One direct result of this project has been that the Alcohol and Drug Abuse Division of the Colorado Department of Health, which is the entity responsible for licensure and contracting with agencies providing substance abuse services, has formally recognized and now provides reimbursement for case management activities.

In addition, through a competitive bidding process, Arapahoe House secured a contract with the aforementioned Division to conduct a pilot demonstration project targeted at the most chronically debilitated clients. The primary goal for this project is, through intensive dyadic case management, to reduce readmissions to our detoxification program by 75% in the first year. Approximately 325 clients will receive services each year.

The timing of this project is propitious, as it commences during the final stages of the NIAAA project. This has enabled Arapahoe House to retain the Case Manager Coordinator and six case manager positions.

CONCLUSIONS

The fundamental concept for this project was to demonstrate and evaluate an intensive case management model, utilizing dyads of case managers, embedded in a system in which an array of substance abuse services is reasonably available to clients. In a very real sense, this project is contrasting a more traditional continuum of substance abuse treatment services with intensive dyadic case management as an overlay to this continuum. This project was a gratifying experience for a number of reasons. First, it has been an exciting and challenging project for the Arapahoe House and University of Denver staffs, respectively. Second, interacting and exchanging ideas with the principals from thirteen sites across this country has been stimulating and of practical value. Third, a substantial number of homeless people with alcohol or other drug problems received services that, in the absence of this project, simply would not have been available. Fourth, the project has had a positive impact on Colorado, both in terms of an infusion of additional resources and the introduction of intensive case management as a strategy that may be of benefit to this target population.

REFERENCES

Braucht, G. N. & Reichardt, C. S. (In press). A computerized approach to trickle-process random assignment. *Evaluation Review.*

Breakey, W. R. (1987). Treating the homeless. *Alcohol, Health and Research World, 11*(3), 42-46.

Finney, J. & Moos, R. (1989). Theory and method in treatment evaluation. *Evaluation and Program Planning, 12,* 307-316.

Graham, K. & Birchmore-Timney, C. (1989). The problem of replicability in program evaluation. *Evaluation and Program Planning, 12,* 179-187.

Harris, M. & Bachrach, L.L. (1988). Clinical case management. *New Directions for Mental Health Services, 40.*

Kline, J. Harris, M., Bebout, R.R. & Drake, R.E. (1991). Contrasting integrated and linkage models of treatment for homeless, dually diagnosed adults. *New Directions for Mental Health Services, 50,* 95-106.

Miller, W. R. & Hester, R.K. (1986). Matching problem drinkers with optimal treatments. In W.R. Miller & N. Heather (Eds.), *Treating addictive behaviors: Processes of change.* New York: Plenum Press.

National Institute on Alcohol Abuse and Alcoholism. (1991). *Glossary of service activities for alcohol and other drug abuse treatment of Homeless persons.* (Contract No. ADM 281-90-0003 with R.O.W. Sciences, Inc.). Rockville, MD. National Institute on Alcohol Abuse and Alcoholism.

Wittman, F.D. (1987). Alcohol, architecture, and homelessness. *Alcohol, Health and Research World, 11*(3), 74-79.

RELAPSE AND RETENTION: PHILADELPHIA

Retention Issues in Treating Homeless Polydrug Users: Philadelphia

Gerald J. Stahler, PhD
Thomas E. Shipley, PhD
David Bartelt, PhD
Danielle Westcott, MBA
Ellen Griffith, MHA
Irving Shandler, MSW

SUMMARY. The present paper describes client engagement issues encountered in a research demonstration program that provides treat-

---

Dr. Gerald Stahler is Assistant Professor, and Dr. David Bartelt is Associate Professor in the Department of Geography and Urban Studies at Temple University. Dr. Bartelt is also Director of Temple's Institute for Public Policy Studies. Dr. Thomas Shipley is Professor of Psychology at Temple University and Danielle Westcott is Project Director of the Temple/DRC Research Demonstration Project. Irving Shandler is President, and Ellen Griffith is Vice President, of the Diagnostic and Rehabilitation Center of Philadelphia.

[Haworth co-indexing entry note]: "Retention Issues in Treating Homeless Polydrug Users: Philadelphia." Stahler, Gerald J. et al. Co-published simultaneously in the *Alcoholism Treatment Quarterly* (The Haworth Press, Inc.) Vol. 10, No. 3/4, 1993, pp. 201-215; and: *Treatment of the Chemically Dependent Homeless: Theory and Implementation in Fourteen American Projects* (ed: Kendon J. Conrad, Cheryl I. Hultman, and John S. Lyons) The Haworth Press, Inc., 1993, pp. 201-215. Multiple copies of this article/chapter may be purchased from The Haworth Document Delivery Center [1-800-3-HAWORTH: 9:00 a.m. - 5:00 p.m. (EST)].

ment for homeless polydrug users in Philadelphia. To better understand the reasons for premature program disengagement, various points of attrition in the subject recruitment and program sequence were identified, process evaluation data were used to closely monitor attrition, client interviews with program dropouts were conducted, and feedback was solicited from staff. In response to the problem, a multi-pronged strategy was formulated to reduce the number of clients leaving prior to completing treatment, and to increase the number who re-engage with the program.

INTRODUCTION

One of the major challenges confronting programs which attempt to help homeless drug users is maintaining client engagement in treatment. As Breakey (1987) and Shipley, Shandler, and Penn (1989) have described, people who are homeless and addicted to drugs pose particular challenges to treatment because they often suffer from disaffiliation, tend to mistrust treatment institutions, are highly mobile, and present a multiplicity of needs. The present paper describes a research demonstration project located in Philadelphia which seeks to assess the efficacy of three different treatment modalities for men who are homeless and addicted to one or more drugs and alcohol, the problems encountered in maintaining program engagement with these clients, and the programmatic responses that have been made to deal with client attrition.

The population in this study consists primarily of shelter-based homeless African-American males who, in Philadelphia, comprise the majority of the homeless population. According to one recent study based on emergency shelter residents in Philadelphia (Goldstein, Bartelt, & Ryan, 1989), African-American males constituted more than half of the total adult (18-45 year old) homeless population, and represented over 72% of the single homeless population. Philadelphia's homeless are fairly young, with a median age of 31, and nearly 90% are under the age of 45. While there are no definitive data on the prevalence of alcohol and other drug use among this population, Goldstein et al. (1989) found that emergency housing providers cited drug and alcohol use as the dominant non-financial reason for homelessness among single adult minority males. As is the case with most of the nation, Philadelphia has been struggling with how to deal with homeless people in a city that has been undergoing major fiscal crises largely attributable to the city's shift from a manufacturing to a post-industrial city (Adams et al., 1991). Public policy in this arena has shifted frequently as the municipal government has vainly searched for solutions in a resource poor environment. This has impacted greatly upon the homeless because of the instability of funding for services to this population.

Few treatment facilities exist in Philadelphia to attempt to provide services to this special population. Perhaps the best established program in Philadelphia that provides such services is the Diagnostic and Rehabilitation Center of Philadelphia (DRC), which, in conjunction with Temple University, developed the present research demonstration program. The Philadelphia project is a continuation of an enduring partnership between Temple University and DRC which has had a long history of conducting research and providing services for people with alcohol and other drug problems including the homeless. Since the 1960s, DRC has grown from a provider that targeted chronic public inebriates to one that operates a comprehensive treatment program for primarily low-income homeless clients, develops new and innovative programs, and operates the city's largest shelter for homeless men. As a grantee in the first round of the National Institute for Alcohol Abuse and Alcoholism (NIAAA) homeless demonstration initiative, DRC and Temple developed a residential treatment program for homeless women and their children. The present project, as mentioned above, targets homeless men, the population which appears to be the most prevalent and difficult to serve in Philadelphia.

The major thrust of this project involves the comparison of three treatment modalities for men who are homeless, and addicted to one or more drugs and alcohol. Using a true experimental design, the study attempts to randomly assign to one of three treatment conditions over a 16 month intake period 700 adult male research subjects who consent to participate in the project. The three treatment conditions consist of the following: *Group 1*, a 6 month comprehensive, integrated residential treatment program located at two sites owned and operated by the Diagnostic and Rehabilitation Center (DRC); *Group 2*, a 4 to 9 month shelter-based intensive case management program staffed by DRC professional and peer counselors; and *Group 3*, a program of regular shelter services provided by city-staffed case managers. Groups 2 and 3 are both based at the Ridge Avenue Shelter, the largest men's shelter in Philadelphia. The project began serving clients on April 1, 1991. After one year of program operations, a total of 545 clients had entered the study with a median age of 32. Slightly more than 90% are African-American, 6% are white, and less than 2% are Hispanic. Crack cocaine is admitted to be the greatest substance abuse problem for 75% of the clients, and alcohol for about 20%. The average age at which an individual first became homeless is 29 years, and the average length of time homeless is 16 months.

By the end of the study, it is anticipated that 700 men will have been randomly assigned to these three treatment conditions with data collected at baseline, discharge, and six months after discharge. The study is primarily directed toward assessing the effectiveness of these treatment approaches in regard to reducing drug and alcohol use, fostering placement in independent living, increasing employment status, improving family and social relations, and enhancing mental health. In addition, the study will attempt to identify the service utilization patterns that best predict success and failure of treatment for these service delivery models; and attempt to determine what personal factors (demographic, social/psychological) best predict success and failure of treatment.

TREATMENT PROGRAMS

All clients who participate in the project are recruited from the long-term beds of the Ridge Avenue Shelter which is managed by DRC under contract with the city. At the inception of the project, the shelter provided 300 long term beds and 120 one night beds for overnight reception. Because of changes in the funding of the shelter, the number of long term beds was reduced during the first year of the project to 175. Clients with alcohol and substance abuse problems are initially recruited for the study by intake staff. Those who consent to participate are referred to an interviewer within 24 hours for the baseline data collection interview. Following the interview, they are randomly assigned to one of the three treatment groups.

Group 1: Residential Treatment Settings

The program philosophy of the residential treatment setting is essentially that addiction is a life-long disease with profound physical, psychological, social, and spiritual consequences for the addicted person, the family, friends, and the community at large. The treatment approach is focused on the addiction, the problems relating to that addiction, and the process of recovery. The therapeutic techniques employed are tailored to the specific needs of each client. "Anchor" counselors assume the responsibility for the treatment process through individual and group counseling, and coordinate all of the services provided to their clients on-site. They provide encouragement and support, and act as positive role models. Through the therapeutic relationship established with staff as well as with other clients, the client learns to accept the fact that he has an illness, the nature of the illness, and the problems it has created. Further, clients learn about the "mechanics" of sobriety, and how to assume responsibility for their own recovery and life style. DRC views twelve-step programs as one of the most effective means of maintaining sobriety, and to this end, it has AA and NA meetings on the premises and encourages participation as the keystone of a lifetime recovery process.

The program provides individualized therapeutic treatment through individual counseling, group therapy, and lectures. Special interest groups are offered, such as AIDS counseling, relapse prevention, anger management groups, and parenting training. The counselors, who have at a minimum a Baccalaureate degree, develop treatment plans for each client in order to define long and short range goals and design strategies to meet these goals. Periodic case consultations are conducted with counselors on each case. While almost all services and activities are provided at the treatment facility and are targeted at the individual client, counselors in some instances may work with the family and/or friends when appropriate and utilize other community resources as required. However, the predominant treatment philosophy is centered on the individual.

The approximate length of treatment for an individual in this group is six to nine months. DRC considers treatment completed if the client is able to assume most or all of the responsibility for his life in the following key areas: recovery from addiction, stabilized physical health, improved interpersonal relationships, adequate housing, vocational/educational pursuits and income management. The program consists of two phases which occur in two locations. During the first phase of treatment, clients reside for about two months in the 35 bed Intermediate Residence unit. Its primary function is to enable clients to become more stabilized so that effective treatment can take place. Three meals a day, as well as snacks, are provided to residents. Lounge space is available for a variety of leisure-time activities such as reading, TV, games and films. A plan is developed for each resident for their activities on the unit. All therapeutic treatment is provided by anchor counselors who have an average caseload of about 20.

Usually, after two months, the client then enters the second phase of treatment which involves continuing outpatient care at DRC along with the support system of AA/NA, and transfer to a 35 bed transitional living facility called Washington House. The special aspect of Washington House is that it operates in tandem with the outpatient treatment component of DRC. Its purpose is to provide a stabilized, growth-oriented living environment, in conjunction with addiction treatment. Emphasis is placed on gaining employment and establishing independent housing. Clients are offered life skills preparation, job search skills training, vocational and educational training, and help with re-entry into the job market. An important element of this treatment approach is that it requires the individual to make a complete commitment to treatment and sobriety. They must reside in the treatment facilities and devote nearly all of their time and effort to the process of recovery. For example, if they are employed, they must give up their jobs to participate in the program until they are well on their way to recovery.

Group 2: Shelter-Based Intensive Case Management

The Group 2 program follows a somewhat less intensive and less restrictive model in that clients remain in the shelter and receive the services of resource and information specialists (RIS). This unit, which is housed in the shelter, attempts to link each resident with the necessary resources in the city to solve his problems and meet his basic needs. Counseling services are provided by outpatient counselors at DRC as well as at other drug and alcohol treatment facilities in the city.

The RIS philosophy stresses the importance of a healthy physical and emotional lifestyle with the goal of self-sufficiency. These specialists through intensive resource and information development, attempt to secure the proper evaluation, treatment, and supports appropriate for their clients to further sober and independent living. Each RIS worker is the "director" helping to orchestrate every step needed for a client: starting with the interviews needed to determine the necessary services, tracking progress, accessing appropriate agencies, and moving the client along to a healthy lifestyle emotionally and physically.

Incorporated in this resource plan is the accountability of the client. It must be documented that he is using the necessary resources to help himself develop a self sufficient life style. In addition to treatment for substance abuse, areas to be addressed include financial assessment/medical coverage/income assistance; income management; educational and vocational training; health care; mental health care; life skills; housing; specialized services for such issues as domestic violence, criminal or delinquent behavior; supportive services for physical disabilities, AIDS, or other special needs; recreational activities; and miscellaneous other resources to meet the individual needs of each resident as assessed by the RIS worker. Income management is an integral part of this intervention. Every client is required to establish some form of income and save a portion of that income for future use for housing when ready to return to the community. The amount to be saved is decided by the client and his RIS worker. Each client has his own interest earning account in his name. Deposits are made with no option for withdrawal until placement or discharge. This savings procedure is mandatory for all clients.

An important characteristic of the Group 2 RIS unit case managers is that they are indigenous workers who are often themselves involved in the recovery process. These individuals are "street smart" and may more easily relate to this population than the more typically degreed social workers or counselors who are often employed as case managers. The average caseload for each case manager is about 15 clients.

Group 3: Shelter-Based Usual Case Management

Clients assigned to this group receive the usual case management services that have been available to shelter residents prior to the inception of this project. City case managers are responsible for helping clients obtain entitlements, finding jobs and housing, and ultimately, getting them off the caseload. Caseloads are extremely high for case managers, sometimes approaching 70 clients per case manager. Consequently, the amount of time devoted to any individual client is substantially less than in either of the two other groups.

MAINTAINING CLIENT RETENTION

Sources of Attrition

Although we had assumed that client retention would be the major problem confronting a successful implementation of the project, this became a larger problem than we had anticipated. Our assumptions about attrition had been based on DRC's past experiences in serving this population and on our experience in the prior demonstration project (Shandler & Shipley, 1987), mentioned earlier, that established a residential treatment setting for homeless polydrug addicted women with children. The results of that study indicated that lifetime cocaine and alcohol involvement, extremes of mood, and reported number of good friends helped to account for the number of days in the program. The greater the prior substance abuse, the longer the stay; the more extreme the negative and positive mood scores and the greater the number of reported good friends, the shorter the stay.

Loss of clients from this project has occurred at the following points in the subject recruitment and program sequence:

1. After consenting to participate, but prior to program assignment (and therefore prior to the baseline assessment point).
2. After assignment to treatment group, but prior to program entry.
3. After entry into program, but prior to completing treatment.

Monitoring Attrition

It became apparent early in the implementation of the project that a key process evaluation activity would be the monitoring of the project's client census and client flow. A specific database was created to monitor client status throughout the life of the project. Included in this database is a comprehensive picture of the sequence of client flow from initial screening for eligibility at the subject recruitment stage, to the number of clients receiving follow-up interviews. These data are presented in a Client Flow Report to the project Steering Committee on a bi-weekly basis. This committee, comprised of the senior program and research staff, represents the project's major oversight and managerial decision-making structure. Virtually all common project concerns are brought to this meeting for discussion and resolution.

During the planning of the project, we had anticipated that approximately 50% of the sample would not complete the experimental treatment programs. After one year of program implementation, a total of 1331 shelter residents had been screened, and 615 had been found to meet the eligibility requirements and had consented to participate. Of this latter group, 545 clients actually received baseline interviews and had been assigned to the three treatment groups.

The first source of attrition, dropping out after providing consent but prior to the baseline interview, has been about 10% during the first year. The second point of attrition, after assignment to treatment group, but prior to program entry, has resulted in a loss of about 17% of those who received baseline interviews. However, nearly all of these clients (90%) had been assigned to Group 1, the setting which provides the most intensive treatment and which has the most restrictive living environment.

Finally, approximately 58% of the client population who had actually entered the two experimental treatment programs (Groups 1 and 2) left prior to completion of their respective experimental treatment programs. These figures include clients who were dismissed for relapse, rule violations, late discovery of ineligibility, as well as those who dropped out of their own accord. For Group 1, program completion consists of abstinence during the six months in residence. For Group 2, completion is defined on an individual basis by a case consultation team. Generally, criteria for completion in this treatment group includes active involvement in recovery services (including outpatient counseling and regular attendance at AA and NA meetings), demonstrated ability to pay rent and save money for future needs, and independent living. For Group 3 clients, there is no formal program completion. About 90% of the clients in this group have left the shelter and are no longer receiving case management services at the site.

In response to these data, the Steering Committee decided to attempt to ascertain the reasons for attrition so as to develop solutions to this project implementation barrier. In addition to continuing to carefully monitor client status, the following three approaches were initiated to find out what was causing the high attrition rates:

1. Informally assessing the reasons for program disengagement based on discussions with program staff;
2. Carefully reviewing the extant process and client flow data in a more refined way to better understand the reasons for dropout–that is, examining various types of attrition for each treatment group;
3. Conducting semi-structured interviews with a sample of 35 clients who had disengaged (which is more than 10% of that population) to ask them about the reasons for their discontinuance in treatment programs;
4. Analyzing baseline data to determine whether dropouts differ from non-dropouts.

Reasons for Attrition

While it is impossible to quantify them precisely, a number of reasons for disengagement from treatment programs were identified. The first reason stems from our recruitment site. We have drawn our sample from a shelter population. Most of these men have come to the shelter for lodging and are not necessarily at that moment concerned or interested in substance abuse treatment. Obtaining treatment is often only of secondary concern to many of our clients. In addition, because clients are recruited so early in their shelter stay, many are quite dysfunctional. Sometimes this has been reflected in the numerous administrative discharges that occur within the first couple of weeks after program entry when many clients are asked to leave the program for a variety of reasons, including curfew violations, altercations with staff or other clients, relapse, or a general disinclination toward maintaining sobriety and "staying clean." A number of clients were unable to tolerate waiting periods for program entry caused by delays in receiving medical assistance approval, or insufficient bed space. This was particularly applicable to Group 1 which has a limited capacity for bed space.

A lack of fit between a client's preferred treatment modality and his assigned treatment group has also been problematic. Unfortunately, this is unavoidable in a study where clients are randomly assigned to three very different types of treatment modalities. Clients who left treatment often reported the restrictiveness, pressure, and structure of the treatment milieu as being major precipitants for their departure. While this was relevant to all three groups, it was particularly mentioned as a problem for clients assigned to Group 1 who must give up jobs and outside contact during the initial phase of treatment. Similarly, the sense of restrictiveness was also manifested in the perceptions of staff whom some clients believed to be overly authoritarian. Conversely, some clients assigned to Group 3 stated that the program was not sufficiently intensive nor structured.

Finally, there were a number of external factors that may have influenced the clients' decision to leave treatment. Some clients wished to return to their girlfriends, friends, or family members. A few wished to return to jobs or trade school. Interviews with these individuals suggested that these reasons often worked in tandem with other reasons such as a lack of readiness for treatment or a dislike for the structured environment of the residential treatment setting.

The Response: Strategies for Reducing Attrition and Increasing Re-Engagement

A subcommittee of the project's Steering Committee was formed for the sole purpose of examining the issue of attrition and making programmatic recommendations on how to reduce subject loss and how to increase treatment re-engagement. In general, the overall strategy was a multi-pronged approach which included reducing the number of ineligible clients who begin the program in the first place; making group-specific programmatic changes, particularly targeting the transitions within the programmatic sequence since these were known to be periods of high attrition; improving re-engagement by enhanced follow-up efforts; and introducing an aftercare program to clients while they are still residing in their respective treatment programs.

Group 1 Initiatives. For Group 1 specifically, one of the major concerns was the nearly 50% loss of clients between assignment to Group 1 and program entry. As mentioned earlier, much of this may be due to the fact that many men simply do not wish to be in such a structured and restrictive treatment program. On the other hand, a number of men would leave the program while they waited for a bed to open at DRC. In response to the men leaving while on the waiting list, several strategies were attempted to maintain the client's interest in the program, ease his transition from a shelter environment to the more structured residential treatment setting, and to improve his readiness for treatment. Men assigned to Group 1 who were waiting for a bed were invited to attend daily orientation sessions at DRC's main treatment facility until placement could be secured. A peer engagement system which matches a successful resident of the program with a new "recruit" from the shelter was set up. In addition, immediately after assignment to Group 1, clients were given a tour of the DRC main facility and Washington House by a case manager. The objective of the tour was to reduce anxiety about the unknown and give the individual concrete information by which to judge the merits of waiting for treatment. This was also to help correct any erroneous preconceived notions about the treatment facility based on rumor or word-of-mouth. Some delays in entering Group 1 treatment were also caused by waiting for a medical assistance card. To remedy this problem, DRC was able to obtain emergency medical assistance cards valid for 30 days from the Department of Public Assistance. Clients could then begin receiving services at DRC rather than having to wait for the arrival of their medical assistance cards.

Finally, a new screening procedure was introduced at intake to reduce the number of clients who were discharged from Group 1 because of a post-placement discovery of ineligibility due to prior rule violations. These cases would therefore represent administrative errors in sampling and would have to be excluded from our analyses. Before receiving a baseline interview, clients were screened for eligibility by the Group 1 program coordinator who maintains a list of program participants who have been discharged for rule violations. In general, while there was a high number of administrative discharges for rule violations, this has not as yet prompted program management to reconsider the rule structure for this setting. This is because most of the rules violations concerned substance use, refusal of payment, or altercations with staff or clients and the enforcement of these rules are seen as consistent with the treatment philosophy as well as necessary to maintain the stability of the setting.

Group 2 Initiatives. For Group 2, it was assumed that the marginal living conditions at the shelter had contributed to client attrition. The shelter atmosphere was not conducive to harmonious living, especially when coupled with hours of idleness. It is particularly difficult to remain clean and sober when bored and unhappy. Therefore, program retention strategies focused on (1) developing additional recreational and group activities to create a greater sense of "community," and (2) enhancing the physical environment to provide a warmer atmosphere. To create a greater sense of community, Group 2 clients were placed in one contiguous section of the shelter, and evening self-help meetings were initiated. Staff-supervised daily community meetings were instituted to provide information, increase group cohesiveness, and provide a forum for solving problems among members.

Furthermore, a number of recreational activities were launched, including bi-weekly sober dances chaperoned by program staff, a weekly movie night with a television and VCR, board games available on a "check out" basis, evening reading and writing seminars, and weekly Spanish lessons. In addition, the project arranged for the use of a local Salvation Army's recreational facilities for regular basketball games and weightlifting exercise, and weekly and group activities such as bowling and field trips. In addition, a new waiting area was set up which contained comfortable furniture and a small library to provide a warmer atmosphere for welcoming new intakes as well as for use by the current clientele.

Aftercare Program. Perhaps the most important retention as well as re-engagement strategy for both Groups 1 and 2 is the implementation of an aftercare program. In response to the need for sober support, monitoring after treatment, and relapse prevention, a community care caseworker position was created to develop an aftercare program. The purpose of the program has been to provide a supportive link with the client after his primary phase of drug and alcohol treatment is completed. This program component assumes that recovery is a process which may include relapse and the need for re-engagement in treatment. A written planning process for aftercare begins at least one month before completion of Group 1's treatment program, and is ongoing in Group 2. The aftercare program particularly focuses on employment and housing, transition groups which address the anxieties and problems which confront clients as they move toward independent living, crisis intervention and advocacy services, and relapse/re-engagement groups to deal with client feelings associated with relapse.

Re-Engagement at Follow-Up. Finally, the last strategy to reduce program attrition for all groups has been to systematically look for dropouts for follow-up interview purposes and attempt to encourage them to return to treatment. The project has begun to focus considerable attention on encouraging clients who have left their treatment programs prematurely and who have been contacted for follow-up interviews to recommit themselves to recovery and to "re-engage" with their original treatment groups. As efforts increase toward locating clients for follow-up interviews, it is hoped that an increasing number of clients will re-engage in treatment.

DISCUSSION

As we approach the third and final year of this experiment, we are uncertain as to how successful our efforts will prove in improving our program retention rates. Even at the present point in time, however, a number of conclusions have emerged. First, our experience underscores the need, especially in new programs, for active utilization of process evaluation data to monitor program implementation and attrition. Without examining these data, we would not have had adequate information for proposing programmatic changes. These data were of two kinds–quantitative and qualitative. The quantitative data portray our client flow and show the general parameters of concern. The qualitative information garnered from formal interviews with clients as well as informal discussions with staff to some extent explains these quantitative findings. More importantly, the qualitative information suggests interventions to rectify problems. These data would be useless, however, without a program management structure that is committed to problem-solving, and a program management team that has the will, ability, and authority to alter and adapt programs in response to this information.

Second, our experience thus far suggests that the strategies employed to increase client engagement and retention must be tailored to the specific program context and the particular attrition source. The strategies for Group 1 were targeted at reducing the attrition during the transition period between when clients are assigned to the residential treatment center and when they actually begin the program. There have been relatively few changes directed toward actually changing the Group 1 treatment program to increase retention. For Group 2, on the other hand, all the changes were directed toward enhancing the program itself so as to retain more clients in treatment since there is very little subject loss between assignment to group and program entry. For both groups, there has been considerable effort expended toward re-engaging those who have left prior to program completion.

Finally, we must acknowledge that no matter how we change or redesign our programs, there will most likely be a substantial number of clients who do not complete our treatment programs. This is partly because of the severity and multitude of problems that these men present, and also because of our locus of recruitment. In contrast to many programs which recruit clients from drug treatment centers, our project draws upon a pool of men who seek shelter, not necessarily drug treatment. The motivation, and perhaps the requisite readiness to make a major life change may be less on average compared to other homeless, substance abusing populations drawn from other settings. Many men may voluntarily consent to participate in the project without truly understanding the consequences of the decision. The demand characteristics of the recruitment situation may result in those who consent to participate but who really are not ready to commit to treatment. Added to this situation is random assignment to three very different treatment modalities which takes no account of client desires or preferences. It is therefore quite understandable why there is a high rate of clients leaving prior to completing the treatment programs, regardless of the quality of the services. On the other hand, there may also be some clients who are functioning quite well and feel that they do not need treatment, as has been found among psychotherapy dropouts (e.g., Stahler & Eisenman, 1987).

At the completion of our data collection, one of our project's goals is to explore *post hoc* the types of treatment methods that seemed to work best with various types of individuals, as well as which treatment methods did not work or were contraindicated for various types of individuals. As we learn more about how best to help homeless drug addicted people toward recovery and independent living, it may be possible to begin initiating prospective treatment matching studies which take better account of an individual's unique needs, preferences, and characteristics. Perhaps only when we have arrived at that stage in program development and formulation will attrition from treatment be of lesser magnitude.

AUTHOR'S NOTE

The authors would like to acknowledge the contributions of a number of individuals who helped in the preparation of this manuscript and who are currently helping conduct this project. Dr. Eric Cohen provided oversight and analysis of client interviews. Tom O'Malley and Rick Shandler helped formulate and implement programmatic changes to increase client engagement. Alan Fink has maintained the client flow database. In addition, we acknowledge the efforts of our research assistants who have carried out the research: Adonijah Bakari, Deborah Barron, Patricia Dixon, Myra Elder, Dorothy Franzone, Mosi Kamau, Obidike Kamau, Susanna Nemes, Merrie Reig, and Anne Weinberg.

Funding for this project was provided by cooperative research grant number AA08802-03 from the National Institute of Alcoholism and Alcohol Abuse, U.S. Department of Health and Human Services.

Address correspondence to: Dr. Gerald Stahler, Department of Geography and Urban Studies, Gladfelter Hall, Temple University, Philadelphia, PA 19122.

REFERENCES

Adams, C., Bartelt, D., Elesh, D., Goldstein, I., Kleniewski, N., Yancey, W. (1991). *Philadelphia: Neighborhoods, division, and conflict in postindustrial city.* Philadelphia: Temple University Press.

Breakey, W. (1987). Treating the homeless. *Alcohol Health and Research World, 11,* 42-47.

Goldstein, I., Bartelt, D., & Ryan, P. (1989). *Homelessness in Philadelphia: Roots, realities, and resolutions.* Philadelphia, PA: Institute for Public Policy Studies, Temple University and the Philadelphia Committee for the Homeless.

Shandler, I., & Shipley, T. (1987). New focus for an old problem: Philadelphia's response to homelessness. *Alcohol Health and Research World*, Spring, 54-57.

Shipley, T., Shandler, I., & Penn, M. (1989). Treatment and research with homeless alcoholics. *Contemporary Drug Problems*, Fall, 505-526.

Stahler, G., & Eisenman, R. (1987). Psychotherapy dropouts: Do they have poor psychological adjustment? *Bulletin of the Psychonomic Society, 23*, 198-200.

TRANSITION TO INDEPENDENCE: BIRMINGHAM

Comparing Two Substance Abuse Treatments for the Homeless: The Birmingham Project

James M. Raczynski, PhD
Joseph E. Schumacher, PhD
Jesse B. Milby, PhD
Max Michael, MD
Molly Engle, PhD
Maggie Lerner, MSW
Tom Woolley, PhD

James M. Raczynski, Joseph E. Schumacher, Jesse B. Milby, Molly Engle, and Maggie Lerner are affiliated with the Behavioral Medicine Unit, Division of General and Preventive Medicine, University of Alabama School of Medicine, and Department of Health Behavior, School of Public Health, University of Alabama at Birmingham. Max Michael is affiliated with Birmingham Health Care for the Homeless Coalition. Tom Woolley is affiliated with the Department of Biostatistics and Biomathematics, School of Public Health, University of Alabama at Birmingham.

[Haworth co-indexing entry note]: "Comparing Two Substance Abuse Treatments for the Homeless: The Birmingham Project." Raczynski, James M. et al. Co-published simultaneously in the *Alcoholism Treatment Quarterly* (The Haworth Press, Inc.) Vol. 10, No. 3/4, 1993, pp. 217-233; and: *Treatment of the Chemically Dependent Homeless: Theory and Implementation in Fourteen American Projects* (ed: Kendon J. Conrad, Cheryl I. Hultman, and John S. Lyons) The Haworth Press, Inc., 1993, pp. 217-233. Multiple copies of this article/chapter may be purchased from The Haworth Document Delivery Center [1-800-3-HAWORTH: 9:00 a.m. - 5:00 p.m. (EST)].

217

SUMMARY. The Birmingham Comparative Substance Abuse Treatments for the Homeless is a cooperative effort between the Birmingham Health Care for the Homeless Coalition (BHCHC) and investigators at the University of Alabama at Birmingham (UAB). This treatment program provides and compares usual care with enhanced services to homeless persons with substance abuse disorders. The study's aims are to: (1) identify homeless persons with substance abuse problems; (2) provide medical evaluation, observation, and stabilization services; (3) randomly assign at least 150 homeless substance abusers to either a usual care or enhanced day treatment intervention; and (4) evaluate the differential effectiveness of the interventions in reducing alcohol and/or drug use, increasing levels of shelter and residency, and enhancing economic and employment status.

INTRODUCTION

A high prevalence of alcohol abuse, alcoholism, and other substance abuse disorders is found consistently among homeless persons. Prevalence estimates for substance abuse disorders among the homeless range from 20% to 63% (Alabama Department of Public Health, 1992; George, Price, Hauth, Barnette, & Preston, 1991; NIDA, 1989, 1991) with averages ranging between 20% and 35%. Once more, it is apparent that state-of-the-art treatment for substance abuse, which does not address unique problems of concurrent homelessness, is ineffectual. In the only controlled study of substance abuse intervention for a subsample of homeless, 100% dropped from the program before treatment was completed (O'Brien, Alterman, Walter, Childress, & McLellan, 1989). Whether substance abuse is viewed as a cause or consequence of homelessness, these data clearly highlight the need for investigation of methods to provide unique substance abuse treatment targeted for homeless persons.

There are a number of unique problems among homeless substance abusers, which suggest the structure of treatment programs needed to address these problems. High co-morbidity rates of physical (Coulehan, Zettler-Segal, Black, McClelland, & Schulberg, 1987; Kamerow, Pincus, & Macdonald, 1986; Weisner & Schmidt, 1992) and mental disorders (Sokol, Martier, & Ager, 1989) in substance abusing homeless persons suggest the potential for increased disability and extended treatment needs (Dever, Kalsbeek, & Sanders, 1992; Goodwin & Gause, 1991; Hoegerman, Wilson, Thurmond, & Schnoll, 1990; NIDA, 1989; Regier, Myers, & Kramer, 1984; Williams, Stinson, Parker, Harford, & Noble, 1987), emphasizing the need to present substance abuse services within broader medical and mental health treatment contexts. The risk of transmission of the HIV

virus and tuberculosis infection in public shelters presents unique management problems from both medical and social perspectives (Daghestani,
1988). Needs of the homeless family are a factor which must be addressed
(Connolly & Marshall, 1991). Increasing awareness of the availability of
services and enhancing access and coordination of these services are critical
issues (Kessei et al., 1984; Roth, Bean, & Hyde, 1986). There is also a
critical need to address housing and vocational and job training among
homeless persons. These multiple factors indicate the multi-faceted nature
of substance abuse disorders among the homeless and the need for a multi-
dimensional treatment approach which coordinates and enhances use of a
range of community services to effectively reach and treat this population
(Dever, Kalsbeek, & Sanders, 1992; Frances, 1988; Gelberg & Linn, 1989;
Gelberg, Linn, & Leake, 1988; NIDA, 1989; Ropers & Boyer, 1987).

The Birmingham Comparative Substance Abuse Treatments Among
the Homeless Project is being conducted as a cooperative effort between
investigators at the University of Alabama at Birmingham (UAB) and at
the Birmingham Health Care for the Homeless Coalition (BHCHC). The
purpose of this paper is to describe the multi-faceted program that has been
developed and that addresses a comparison of usual care to an enhanced day
treatment program for substance abusing homeless, a treatment involving
vocational and social training, and renovation of drug-free housing for
successfully rehabilitated clients.

BACKGROUND OF THE BIRMINGHAM PROJECT

The Birmingham Comparative Substance Abuse Treatments for the
Homeless Project was funded by the National Institute on Alcoholism and
Alcohol Abuse and the National Institute on Drug Abuse as one of 14
demonstration projects across the country to study substance abuse treatments
among the homeless. The Birmingham Project was conceptualized and remains
a cooperative effort between staff at the BHCHC and faculty at UAB. In this
effort, BHCHC functions as the service provider, recruiting participants and
providing both project-designed usual care and enhanced services to the
homeless participants. Faculty from UAB serve two major functions in the
project: (1) as a resource for professional consultation and support in implementing the program; and (2) as the members of the investigative team that
provide the scientific expertise for the project, including expertise in the
design, implementation, and conduct of the project's evaluation.

Setting

Prior to implementing the comparative programs of this project in May,
1991, BHCHC provided direct health care and social services to 2,300

homeless persons through more than 12,000 patient encounters in 1989. Of those seen, more than 38 percent of the clients had a diagnosis of alcohol abuse while an additional 13 percent had a diagnosis of abusing substances other than alcohol. Although skeletal and limited in scope, BHCHC offered a range of counseling and case management services to clients with substance abuse disorders.

Participants are recruited for the project from those clients seeking services at BHCHC, and eligibility, baseline, and follow-up evaluations of participants are conducted at a central site by trained and certified interviewers. The treatment programs for the project are conducted at two other treatment sites with one program (either usual care or enhanced care) being offered at each site. Conducting the programs in two separate locations minimizes concerns about contamination between the interventions, at least during the time when participants are involved in the program. All data management, data entry, and data storage for the project are conducted in office space at UAB, located within approximately three miles of both BHCHC treatment facilities. UAB project staff, including investigators, research interviewers, and data management personnel, are also located in office space at UAB.

Birmingham Homeless Population

The profile of Birmingham, Alabama's homeless persons, derived from previous data collected for the BHCHC in which 150 homeless persons were randomly sampled (LaGory, Ritchey, & Mullins, 1987), is generally consistent with the findings of other national surveys. The Birmingham homeless are predominantly native Alabamians, male (77%), and white (61%) (although street-based homeless were disproportionately black and male), with a mean age of 39.7 years. A majority of those interviewed were found to have diverse and complex constellations of social, psychological, and physical needs which were not being met. A significant portion of those surveyed were found to have their status as homeless either preceded or accompanied by stressful life events, most commonly attributed to job loss (75%), interpersonal problems (60%), or problems of substance abuse (64%).

Characteristics of Project Participants

Basic characteristics for the 178 project participants are: 80.7% are male, 19.3% are female; 8% are white, and 92% are African American; mean age is 31.1 years ($SD = 6.4$) with a range of 21 to 51 years; and mean education is 12.1 years ($SD = 2.0$) with a range of 3 to 20 years. This suggests that project participants were somewhat younger and disproportionately African American and male than the previous random sample. Thirty-five percent of the sample were veterans. Seventy-seven percent of the sample were diagnosed with cocaine dependence (primarily crack cocaine), 47.3% were diagnosed with alcohol dependence, and 6% had diagnoses of cannabis and other unspecified substance abuse disorders. Twenty-six percent of the sample carried co-existing cocaine and alcohol dependence disorders. A significant presence of antisocial, borderline, schizoid, and paranoid personality disorders, and depression and dysthymia were observed. The average Beck Depression score at baseline was 21.8, indicating the presence of moderate to severe depression in the sample.

OBJECTIVES

The five objectives of the project as originally conceptualized include: (1) to identify homeless persons with substance abuse problems through already established outreach methods; (2) to provide medical evaluation and observation services to those identified as potential participants with the provision of acute medical care and stabilization to those individuals needing such intervention; (3) to randomly assign at least 150 identified homeless persons who have alcohol and/or drug problems, who are willing to participate and who provide informed consent over the 15 months of recruitment to either usual care or enhanced day treatment intervention; (4) to provide usual care to those randomized to this intervention, consisting of access to twice weekly substance abuse group treatment and other services normally available to all homeless persons through BHCHC and referral services; and (5) to provide enhanced day treatment intervention for those randomized to this intervention.

The enhanced treatment differs from usual care and customary treatment in several key respects. First, the enhanced care treatment provides a more intensive form of treatment, meeting every weekday for most of the day as opposed to only twice weekly for individual therapy meetings. Second, the enhanced care offers participants a fuller range of treatment services than usual care, addressing the complexity of substance abuse disorders among homeless persons better than usual care. Finally, the integral housing component of the enhanced care differentiates the two forms of treatment. Not only does this component enable integrating vocational training and paid work experience into the treatment program, resulting in systematic success experiences for clients and potential increases in self-esteem, but it results in housing, the potential occupancy of which serves as a reinforcer for clients to remain in the program and achieve success in substance abuse treatment.

PROJECT ORGANIZATION

With a project of this complexity, involving not only the implementation of a complex enhanced intervention, but also the coordination of two organizations with different sets of coordinated activities, one at BHCHC and one at UAB, we believe that a well delineated project organization is essential to ensuring the smooth and efficient functioning of the project. Hence, we have implemented an organizational structure that we believe has facilitated the transfer of information between project staff and the coordination of activities, consisting of three levels of committee structure.

The Executive Committee resides at the highest level of our organizational structure and consists of key investigative and administrative personnel, including the Principal Investigator for the project (Dr. Jesse Milby), the Co-Principal Investigator (Dr. James Raczynski), the Principal Investigator of the sub-contract at BHCHC (Dr. Max Michael, the Medical Director of BHCHC), and Ms. Karen McGee (the Executive Director of BHCHC). The Executive Committee is responsible for overseeing all aspects of the project and making all final decisions concerning the conduct of the project, both programmatic and scientific.

At the next organizational level, the Steering Committee consists of all project staff, including all investigators and staff at both BHCHC and UAB. The Steering Committee is responsible for scientific and operational direction of the study and provides the vehicle through which it is ensured that uniform information is disseminated to all staff. The Steering Committee proposes changes to the Executive Committee who are responsible for making all final decisions regarding the project.

Finally, there are two subcommittees of the Steering Committee: the Program Subcommittee and the Research Committee. The Program Subcommittee consists of the program staff at the BHCHC and the program consultant staff at UAB and is responsible for overseeing the integrity of the enhanced and usual care programs and making program recommendations to the Steering Committee. The Research Committee consists of research investigative personnel at UAB who are responsible for overseeing all evaluation aspects of the project, including data collection and data management, and making research recommendations to the Steering Committee.

ENHANCED DAY TREATMENT

Theoretical Basis for Enhanced Care

The enhanced treatment program is based on the most effective outpatient/day treatment programs for drug and alcohol abusers reported in the literature. Recent programs designed to treat drug abuse, especially co-caine abuse, have found it extremely important to provide daily therapeutic contacts with clients and to quickly intervene both to prevent drug-seeking responses to drug craving, and to focus intervention on helping the drug user find non-drug related pleasurable activities and new sources of non-drug involved socialization (Washton & Stone-Washton, 1990; Wallace, 1991). Learning theory, principles of reinforcement, and animal models research, suggest the efficacy of developing alternative reinforcers and using them to substitute for pharmacological reinforcers. Alternative reinforcers should then strengthen behaviors which compete with drug-seeking. Yet, only one study has approximated this strategy, and it did not treat the more dysfunctional homeless patients and did not systematically use exposure to new reinforcers for all clients (Higgins et al., 1991).

Two effective outpatient interventions for cocaine abuse seem to be emerging from the clinical research: an outpatient/day treatment model like that reported by O'Brien, Alterman, Walter, Childress, and McLellan (1990) and Washton and Stone-Washton (1990) and a contingency management behavioral therapy program with less frequent patient contact (Higgins et al., 1991; Kosten, 1992). The Higgins et al. (1991) study provided subjects with reinforcement contingencies for consecutive clean urines, i.e., sustained abstinence, and counseled subjects to develop new recreational activities or reinvolve themselves with previously enjoyed non-drug related recreational activities. However, none of these programs has reported success with cocaine abusing homeless. O'Brien et al. (1990) reported they were uniformly unsuccessful in treating their homeless cocaine abusers since 100% dropped from the program before completing treatment.

Thus, though no programs have designed interventions for cocaine and alcohol abusing homeless persons, and the one study that included homeless persons was unsuccessful in engaging them in treatment, there seem to be evolving effective outpatient programs for cocaine abuse. Once more, those programs that have reported successful outcome, given reasonable control or comparison conditions (Higgins et al., 1991; O'Brien et al., 1990; Washton & Stone-Washton, 1990), all include common similar elements. Two of the three involve intense daily contact 4-5 days per week (O'Brien et al., 1990; Washton & Stone-Washton, 1990). All involve at least once weekly urine surveillance with feedback to clients and an emphasis on relapse prevention by avoiding old drug using friends and associates and developing new non-drug related sources of gratification, although Higgins et al. (1991) seemed to emphasize this more than the others.

It should be noted that the Birmingham Project was originally conceived for alcoholism intervention and has had to intervene with a patient population with co-existing alcohol and cocaine abuse/dependence and underlying mental illness (mostly Affective and Personality Disorders). Since the literature shows there are successful interventions for cocaine and combined cocaine/alcohol abuse (Higgins et al., 1991; O'Brien, Childress, McLellan, & Ehrman, 1992; Washton & Stone-Washton, 1990), and that contingencies requiring abstinence are effective in other contexts (Milby, Garrett, English, Fritchie, & Clarke, 1978), we incorporated them while at the same time measuring the interactive efficacy of a potentially potent treatment contingency for substance abusing homeless. We studied the impact of abstinence contingent work and housing during the second phase of treatment. By doing so we tested the efficacy of a behavioral social reinforcement approach in the context of a day treatment model, combining the only models for alcohol/cocaine abuse that have some empirical foundation for treatment effectiveness.

Structure of Enhanced Day Treatment

Our multifaceted enhanced treatment program is based on two phases: the day-treatment and the work and housing components. This is a unique combination of substance abuse treatment and work and housing habitation. In addition to creating housing, the benefits of the housing component also accomplish vocational training goals and are expected to result in improvements in clients' overall self-esteem. During the initial two-month day treatment phase, participants are involved in active programming from 7:45 a.m. until approximately 2:00 p.m. every day and remain in residence in shelters or other temporary living arrangements obtained on their own or through the assistance of their counselors. Work and drug-free housing opportunities are made available later on in the project after abstinence is established.

The structure of the first two months of the enhanced day treatment program include: (1) therapeutic community; (2) psychoeducational groups; (3) individualized contract development; (4) individual treatment planning and counseling; and (5) process group therapy. Therapeutic community is a client-governed experience that begins each treatment day. Officers, who are elected monthly, conduct the structured meetings with only a moderating presence by staff who are careful not to usurp the authority of the officers or rescue clients who are struggling with the responsibility of their roles. Therapeutic community meetings provide the foundation for the enhanced treatment experience. A variety of psychoeducational groups are also offered (e.g., relapse prevention, assertiveness training, role play, AIDS awareness, community resources, weekend planning, orientation to housing, relaxation therapy, stress management, 12-steps, and vocational training). Individualized contracts are developed within the first week of treatment and provide goals and specific tasks for each client to implement in various groups, as well as outside the treatment environment. In addition to the structured, psycho-educational nature of the day-treatment program, a strong experiential component exists. Intense sharing of positive and negative experiences and emotions, lending of support and love, confronting denial and "stinkin' thinkin'," and identifying positive behaviors of others creates a cohesive bond among the clients and staff and promotes a therapeutic environment.

After completion of the first two-month day treatment phase and a minimum of two weeks of drug-free test results, clients become eligible for participation in the work and housing components. Activities at this phase are designed to provide on-the-job vocational skill development and paid work experience. Affiliation with Bad Boy Builders, under the direction of a local building contractor (Mr. Jerry Vann), offers a variety of work sites and jobs, including renovation of structures to be occupied by the clients themselves and as drug-free residences for the project. Housing is available to clients who are working and able to pay a modest rent and who remain drug-free and responsible renters. House meetings, in-home AA/NA/CA meetings, and house governments modeled after the Oxford House program are being incorporated into the housing component at clients' requests. Counselors report that the work and housing components of the project are considered to be highly valued by both incoming clients and clients who remain in the program.

Upon completion of both the day treatment and the work and housing phases, clients are able to remain in the drug-free housing provided by the project on a permanent basis. Program-based work experiences are phased out and clients are assisted in obtaining jobs in the community. Clients are encouraged to attend weekly after-care groups which concentrate on relapse prevention, work and shelter maintenance issues.

USUAL CARE TREATMENT

The usual care intervention approximates the standard of usual care available in the community and offered by BHCHC prior to program implementation. During the six months of usual care treatment, clients are seen twice weekly for individual and group counseling by trained substance abuse counselors. Counselors also function as case managers, attempting to access shelter and additional treatment services for clients as appropriate.

IMPLEMENTATION

Four major problems were encountered in the implementation of the project: (1) building a research/service delivery coalition; (2) implementing the complex, multifaceted enhanced treatment program; (3) dealing with community response to the housing component of the enhanced treatment program; and (4) enrollment and tracking of participants. Some individuals acknowledge that conflicts often arise when efforts are made to coordinate service delivery and research activities, although the reasons for these perceptions of conflict may not be based on an actual inherent conflict in research and community needs (Raczynski & Lewis, in press).

Nonetheless, despite our efforts to structure clear and effective lines of communication and to plan carefully our activities, when we began implementing the usual care and enhanced programs, we encountered concerns about the overall structure of activities designated for UAB and BHCHC. Concerns raised between BHCHC and UAB personnel were focused less on the structure of the evaluation activities and more on the extent to which UAB investigators would serve as a source of professional expertise and exert control over the program and BHCHC staff during implementation of the enhanced treatment program. These concerns were addressed in two manners: (1) the Executive Committee clarified more explicitly the roles of investigative and staff personnel at both BHCHC and UAB; and (2) personnel changes were implemented at UAB to ensure that UAB investigative and staff personnel had more frequent and structured contact with BHCHC staff. These personnel changes consisted of: designating Dr. Schumacher, a clinical psychologist, as Program Director (and more recently as Co-Principal Investigator) at UAB, charged with defining the extent and scope of consultative support with the BHCHC staff; and (2) designating a clinical psychology fellow at UAB as a relatively non-threatening professional staff member who was assigned to be present at BHCHC on a daily basis to assist BHCHC staff and model appropriate therapeutic behaviors. It is our belief that the most effective means of overcoming role conflicts between academic and service delivery investigative and staff personnel is implementing a program with clear role definition as well as, and perhaps more importantly, structuring activities in which personnel must work together.

Implementing the complex, multifaceted enhanced treatment program was also a challenge faced by project personnel. Program service delivery staff consist of master's and bachelor's level staff, who have excellent training and experience. However, their experience has not been with programs as complex and extensive as those designed for the enhanced program. Implementation of the enhanced program, therefore, necessitated cooperative efforts between faculty at UAB and project staff at BHCHC. Although a challenge, once the research/service delivery coalition was functioning effectively, the project's organization seemed adequate to coordinate activities and foster the successful implementation of the enhanced program.

Dealing with the community response to the housing component of the enhanced treatment program was somewhat more challenging than other problems encountered during implementation, since this conflict was not internal within the project. As renovation began on the first house, the surrounding community became aware of the project's activities and undertook efforts to block the use of the house by clients. Community response included not only efforts made through legitimate channels to block activities, such as through community petition to City of Birmingham Council Members, but also resulted in vandalism to the property. To address this problem, BHCHC and UAB staff relied on NIAAA consultants for legal and practical advice. Based on this advice, the decision was made to establish a non-profit corporation, Pioneer Systems, that would manage the housing, effectively separating the housing and other service delivery components. While this step may not have altered the perceived threat by community residents from having homeless persons move into housing in the neighborhood, it did disentangle issues concerning housing with issues involving other services, including the substance abuse treatment programs, offered by BHCHC. Legally, the Fair Housing Act ensures equal access to housing, and this point was also addressed with City of Birmingham officials. Whether these steps were effective or community attention was diverted from housing for other reasons, the controversy that arose from housing ameliorated as the project progressed.

The final major problem encountered was that of enrolling and tracking a sufficient number of participants. As might be anticipated, enrollment of participants was relatively easy during periods of inclement weather. However, during periods in which the weather was not very cold (which is most months except December and January in Birmingham), enrollment was slow. Early problems were encountered in implementing the housing component, partly due to problems encountered with the community as we have discussed, and not budgeting within project funds to pay participants for their work doing renovation as part of the housing component. Originally, project investigators and staff conceptualized the renovation work as part of the treatment program and, as such, activity that would not result in pay to participants. However, as participants quickly noted, their involvement in renovation prohibited their making money through other means, such as collecting and selling aluminum cans. Knowledge about these problems spread from participants to homeless persons who were prospective participants in Birmingham. To address problems with not paying participants during renovation work, project funds were re-budgeted to ensure that participants could be paid for their work during renovation activities.

To bolster further enrollment, foster a more positive impression of the project, increase attendance, and improve tracking, BHCHC staff proposed that Club Birmingham be implemented for all persons who entered the project. Club activities consist of monthly cook-outs, ID cards, raffles for regular attendance, and other benefits (such as distribution of sweat shirts and hats emblazoned with the Club Birmingham logo to all enrollees). These activities resulted in an increase in enrollment and final randomization of the expected number of participants.

Problems have also been encountered with tracking participants for follow-up assessments. Initial efforts to follow clients after treatment consisted of a fifteen dollar incentive and a pocket calendar with follow-up assessment dates. We found early on that these strategies were simplistic and ineffective. The first signs of increased follow-up rates resulted from the efforts of Club Birmingham. Recently, we have implemented a complex and integrated tracking plan based on the work of one of our sister projects in New Orleans, that utilizes one full-time tracker and two part-time "client" trackers representing the usual care and day treatment programs. These staff are engaged in mail, phone, agency, shelter, and street tracking activities.

Despite these problems, the project has been implemented as originally proposed, with two very different treatment programs. The consensus of project evaluation personnel has been that both clients as well as staff at BHCHC are well aware of the discrepancies in services between usual care and the enhanced treatment approaches even though the participants and staff in the two programs are physically separated from one another. To an evident degree, the consensus is that both clients and staff in the usual care program are demoralized with the perception that the enhanced day treatment program offers a greater number of services than are provided in usual care. Current efforts to assess the nature and extent of the demoralization, through the administration of the Community-Oriented Programs Environment Scale (Moos, 1987) to all present clients and staff and at 6-month follow-up, are underway.

As with most community research programs, an area of critical concern for project personnel has been the continuation of services at the end of the grant period. While some components of the enhanced program, e.g., the day treatment activities, will require funding to continue, other aspects, e.g., drug-free housing will be able to continue with relatively little, if any, outside funding. While it is too early to project all of the costs of the housing activities, we anticipate, with the continuing source of assets accrued from rent of housing, that enough money may be accumulated to cover the minimal costs for leasing and purchase of HUD and even non-HUD housing and the renovation of this housing. This approach to housing is obviously predicated on the availability of suitable housing stock for lease or purchase, and this suitable housing may not be available everywhere. However, in places, such as Birmingham, where suitable housing is plentiful, this approach may be replicable.

PRELIMINARY FINDINGS

Since enrolling the first client in April, 1991, through July 30, 1992, a total of 176 clients have been enrolled and randomized to either usual care (87 participants) or enhanced treatment (89 participants). This number exceeded our original recruitment goal of 150 participants. Comparisons between usual care and enhanced treatment groups suggest no differences at baseline between the groups on key demographic and descriptive variables including: age, race, length of time homeless, use of substances, shelter and employment variables.

Preliminary results of key substance abuse, depression, self-esteem, and situational confidence outcome variables across two time periods (baseline to 2-month and baseline to 6-month) have been compiled as percent increases and percent decreases. Comparisons between usual care and day treatment groups suggested no significant differences on key demographic and outcome variables at baseline. Findings suggest that both usual care and day treatment had an impact on key outcome variables at the baseline to 2-month period. For usual care, decreases in substance use ranged from 33.3 percent to 60.5 percent. However, for day treatment, decreases in substance use were greater than usual care and ranged from 63.8 percent to 87.1 percent. At the 6-month period, usual care showed increases in alcohol, marijuana, and cocaine substances as large as three times the use at baseline. For day treatment, alcohol use increased by 17.5 percent, but marijuana use decreased by 46 percent and cocaine decreased by 62.9 percent. Self-reported problems with alcohol decreased for both usual care and day treatment groups at the baseline to 2-month period. At the baseline to 6-month period, self-reported alcohol and drug problems increased for usual care, but decreased for day treatment. Symptoms of depression decreased for both treatment groups at both assessment points, with fewer symptoms present in the day treatment group. Self-esteem increased in both groups across both time periods, with day treatment doing slightly better at raising self-esteem than usual care. Situational confidence at dealing with drug and alcohol high risk situations increased for both groups across both time periods, with greater confidence revealed in the day treatment group. Employment and housing status are expected to reveal better outcomes in the day treatment group due to the nature of the day treatment, work and housing components. We feel these preliminary findings indicate the efficacy of a day treatment program as it relates to the selected substance use, depression, self-esteem, and situational confidence variables.

IMPLICATIONS FOR PRACTICE AND RESEARCH

Although the project is ongoing, with final one-year follow-up data collection to begin during June, 1993, we believe that there are a number of research and clinical implications that can already be drawn from our experience. Prominent among these implications, we believe that this project is a successful example of the potential for cooperative research endeavors between academic and service delivery institutions. Although this implication may, to some degree be perceived as self-evident, perceptions of inherent incompatibilities and associated conflicts between research activities and community service programs are prominent (Raczynski & Lewis, in press). We encountered these problems, and while they were not easy to overcome, we were able to address them by anticipating them and ensuring that there was an organizational structure to the project capable of dealing with these problems when they occurred. As a demonstration of the extent to which we have been able to overcome these barriers to research/service delivery collaboration, we are now discussing future grant applications to support other collaborative projects.

From a research perspective, the value of this project has yet to be determined since we are not yet able to completely examine our outcome data. However, we believe that we already have data that strongly suggest the benefit of the enhanced program over the usual care program in addressing the multiple needs of substance-abusing homeless persons.

From a clinical perspective, we strongly believe that the implementation of the multi-faceted enhanced program, particularly with the incorporation of the work and housing components with the day-treatment program, may provide a model service delivery program capable of implementation elsewhere. The underlying theoretical assumptions of this project are that substance abuse among homeless persons is a multi-faceted problem requiring a multi-faceted treatment approach. We believe that the complexity of treatment issues may be somewhat greater among homeless persons, who have fewer financial, vocational, and social support resources, than other groups.

Worthy of particular mention is the drug-free housing component of the enhanced treatment program. We believe that this aspect of the overall program addresses four important areas: (1) it clearly is a means of creating suitable housing for homeless clients; (2) it provides vocational training and paid work experience for enhanced treatment clients; (3) it provides a source of immediate success experiences for enhanced treatment clients, increasing self-esteem; and (4) it provides a reward for clients to remain in treatment, since only clients who complete treatment and remain drug-free are eligible for the housing. Of major significance also is the fact that with available, suitable housing stock, this component, once established may be financially self-supporting. Certainly, this component may provide a model for similar programs in areas where there is suitable housing for lease or purchase.

The final evaluation of the Birmingham Comparative Substance Abuse Treatments for the Homeless Project must await analysis of our outcome data in 1993. However, we anticipate that this quantitative and qualitative evaluation will support preliminary data that suggest the benefits of an enhanced treatment program for substance-abusing homeless persons.

AUTHOR'S NOTE

This research was supported by grant AA08819-01 from the National Institute on Alcoholism and Alcohol Abuse and National Institute on Drug Abuse.

LITERATURE CITED

Alabama Department of Public Health. *A Report on the 1991 Alabama Behavioral Risk Factor Survey.* Office of Health Promotion and Information, Health Promotion Branch, Montgomery, AL 1992.

Brady, K. T. (1992). Gender differences in substance abuse: Training issues. *Substance Abuse, 13*(2), 51-52.

Chasnoff, I. J., Landress, H. J., & Barrett, M. E. (1990). The prevalence of illicit drug or alcohol use during pregnancy and discrepancies in mandatory reporting in Pinellas County, Florida. *New England Journal of Medicine, 322,* 1202-1206.

Connolly, W. B., & Marshall, A. B. (1991). Drug addiction, pregnancy, and childbirth: Legal issues for the medical and social services communities. *Clinics in Perinatology, 18*(1), 147-186.

Coulehan, J. L., Zettler-Segal, M., Black, M., McClelland, M., & Schulberg, H. C. (1987). Recognition of alcoholism and substance abuse in primary care patients. *Archives of Internal Medicine, 147*, 349-352.

Daghestani, A. N. (1988). Psychosocial characteristics of pregnant women addicts in treatment. In I. J. Chasnoff (Ed.), *Drugs, alcohol, pregnancy and parenting* (pp. 7-16). Boston: Kluwer Academic Publishers.

Dever, J., Kalsbeek, W., & Sanders, L. (1992). Counseling practices of primary-care physicians–North Carolina, 1991. *Morbidity and Mortality Weekly Report, 41*(31), 565-568.

Frances, R. J. (1988). Update on alcohol and drug disorder treatment. *Journal of Clinical Psychiatry, 49*(Suppl), 13-17.

Gelberg, L., Linn, L. S., & Leake, B. D. (1988). Mental health, alcohol and drug use, and criminal history among homeless adults. *American Journal of Psychiatry, 145*, 191-196.

Gelberg, L., & Linn, L. S. (1989). Psychological distress among homeless adults. *Journal of Nervous and Mental Disorders, 177*, 291-295.

George, S. K., Price, J., Hauth, J. C., Barnette, D. M., & Preston, P. (1991). Drug abuse screening of childbearing-age women in Alabama public health clinics. *American Journal of Obstetrics and Gynecology, 165*(4), 924-927.

Goodwin, F. K., & Gause, E. M. (1991). From the Alcohol, Drug Abuse, and Mental Health Administration. *Journal of the American Medical Association, 265*(12), 1510.

Higgins, S., Delaney, D., Budney, A., Bickel, W. K., Hughes, J. R., Foerg, F., & Fenwick, J. W. (1991). A behavioral approach to achieving initial cocaine abstinence. *American Journal of Psychiatry, 148*(9), 1218-1224.

Hoegerman, G. S., Wilson, C. A., Thurmond, E., & Schnoll, S. H. (May, 1990). Drug exposed neonate, in addiction medicine. *Western Journal of Medicine, 152*, 559-564.

Kamerow, D. B., Pincus, H. A., & Macdonald, D. I. (1986). Alcohol abuse, other drug abuse, and mental disorders in medical practice: Prevalence, costs, recognition, and treatment. *Journal of the American Medical Association, 255*(15), 2054-2057.

Kessei, N., Makeniuola, J. D., Rossaii, C. J., Chand, T. G., Hore, B. D., Redmont, A. D., Reen, D. W., Gordon, M., & Wallace, P. C. (1984). The Manchester detoxification service: Description and evaluation. *Lancet, 12*, 839-842.

Kosten, T. (June, 1992). Diverse pharmacological agents for possible treatment of cocaine dependency. *Paper presented at the 54th annual scientific meeting of the College on Problems of Drug Dependence*, Keystone, Colorado.

La Gory, M., Ritchey, F. J., & Mullis, J. (1987). The homeless of Alabama: Preliminary report of the homeless enumeration and survey project. Unpublished manuscript.

Milby, J. B., Garrett, C., English, C., Fritchie, O., & Clarke, C. (1978). Take-home methadone: Contingency effects on drug-seeking and productivity of narcotic addicts. *Addictive Behavior, 3*, 215-220.

Moos, R. H. (1987). *The social climate scales: A user's guide.* Palo Alto, CA: Consulting Psychologists Press, Inc.

National Institute on Drug Abuse, Division of Epidemiology and Prevention Research. (1991). *National household survey on drug abuse: Main findings 1990.* Rockville, MD: U.S. Department of Health and Human Services.

National Institute on Drug Abuse. (1989). *Drug abuse and pregnancy.* U.S. Department of Health and Human Services; 1-4, C-89-04.

O'Brien, C. D., Childress, A. R., McLellan, A. T. & Ehrman, R. (1992). A learning model of addiction. In C. P. O'Brien, & J. H. Jaffe (Eds.). *Addictive States.* New York: Raven Press.

O'Brien, C. P., Alterman, A., Walter, D., Childress, A. R., & McLellan, A. T. (1989). Evaluation of treatment for cocaine dependence. *NIDA Research Monograph, 95,* 78-84.

Raczynski, J., and Lewis, B. (in press). Reconciling the multiple scientific and community needs. *Proceedings on Health Behavior Research in Minority Populations: Access, Design, and Implementation.* Washington, DC: National Institute of Health.

Regier, D. A., Myers, J. K., & Kramer, M. E. (1984). The NIMH Epidemiologic Catchment Area: Historical context, major objectives, and study population characteristics. *Archives of General Psychiatry, 41,* 934-941.

Ropers, R. H., & Boyer, R. (1987). Perceived health status among the new urban homeless. *Society of Scientific Medicine, 24,* 669-678.

Roth, E., Bean, G. J., & Hyde, P. S. (1986). Homelessness and mental health policy: Developing an appropriate role for the 1980s. *Community Mental Health Journal, 22,* 203-214.

Sokol, R. J., Martier, S. S. & Ager, J. W. (1989). The T-ACE questions: Practical prenatal detection of risk-drinking. *American Journal of Obstetrics and Gynecology, 160,* 863-870.

Wallace, B. C. (1991). Crack cocaine: What constitutes state of the art treatment? *Journal of Addictive Diseases, 11*(2), 79-95.

Washton, A. M., & Stone-Washton, N. (1990). Abstinence and relapse in outpatient cocaine addicts. *Journal of Psychoactive Drugs, 22*(2), 135-147.

Wechsler, H., Levine, S., Idelson, R.K., Rohman, M., and Taylor, J.O. The Physician's Role in Health Promotion–A Survey of Primary-Care Practitioners. NEJM 1983; 308(2):97-101.

Weisner, C. & Schmidt, L. (1992). Gender disparities in treatment for alcohol problems. *Journal of the American Medical Association, 268*(14), 1872-1876.

Williams, G. D., Stinson, F. S., Parker, D. A., Harford, T. C., & Noble, J. (1987). Demographic trends, alcohol abuse and alcoholism–1985-1995. *Alcohol Health & Research World Epidemiologic Bulletin, 15,* 80-83.

CONCLUSION

Treatment
of the Chemically Dependent Homeless:
A Synthesis

Kendon J. Conrad, PhD
Cheryl I. Hultman, PhD
John S. Lyons, PhD

This concluding chapter synthesizes some of the major themes of this volume. Because of the large amount of material that is presented in this book, some readers will select only those chapters that are of particular interest and will skip the rest. Therefore, we thought it would be useful to readers for us to attempt a synthesis. In doing so, we must sometimes present generalizations whereas the chapters themselves contain rich detail, anecdotes, and refined rationales that are specific to their particular settings and populations. Additionally, we caution readers that our interpretations may not always accurately represent the ideas of some of the authors of the chapters. Although we draw upon their valuable contributions, we take full responsibility for the interpretations and opinions expressed in

[Haworth co-indexing entry note]: "Treatment of the Chemically Dependent Homeless: A Synthesis." Conrad, Kendon J., Cheryl I. Hultman, and John S. Lyons. Co-published simultaneously in the *Alcoholism Treatment Quarterly* (The Haworth Press, Inc.) Vol. 10, No. 3/4, 1993, pp. 235-246; and: *Treatment of the Chemically Dependent Homeless: Theory and Implementation in Fourteen American Projects* (ed: Kendon J. Conrad, Cheryl I. Hultman, and John S. Lyons) The Haworth Press, Inc., 1993, pp. 235-246. Multiple copies of this article/chapter may be purchased from The Haworth Document Delivery Center [1-800-3-HAWORTH: 9:00 a.m. - 5:00 p.m. (EST)].

this concluding chapter. Throughout this synthesis we refer to the chapters by the name of the city with which the project was identified. The names of the cities are provided in the table of contents and the running head of each chapter.

THEORETICAL PERSPECTIVES

When we use the word "theory" in the context of social programs, we mean sets of statements that explain how the programs are intended to work to foster improvement. The statements are not deterministic in nature, but rather they are probabilistic. In other words, they describe how certain characteristics of programs will probably work to bring about certain beneficial changes in certain types of clients. These statements are important because they guide the implementation of the programs. If some of these projects are found to have beneficial effects, program planners will turn to the theories enacted by these projects as guides for future implementation and program improvement.

The theories represented here vary greatly at some times and subtly at others. Readers must read each chapter to appreciate the rich detail that is presented. However, most of the projects hold that it is extremely difficult to help most of the chemically dependent homeless without providing them with a secure, comfortable, and supervised place to live. Secondarily, that place must be supportive of sobriety. The perspectives in this book differ on how long supervised housing should last, but they all imply that supervised housing is desirable to enable resocialization or getting clients "back on their feet." Once this is accomplished, it must be maintained and accompanied by gradual reintegration into life in the community in independent housing. For independence to be maintained, it is necessary to have established an income through employment and/or benefits. Sobriety maintenance usually requires participation in self-help groups and/or ongoing participation in program activities. Therefore, these interventions facilitate the development and ongoing maintenance of a continuum of treatment and recovery services and a spectrum of housing services within their respective communities.

Huebner and Scott (personal communication), in their review of this chapter, provided a somewhat different perspective. They noted that homeless persons with alcohol or other drug abuse problems who comprise the target populations for these projects have problems which exist across multiple domains—health, housing, economics, substance abuse, etc. Given the multiple and varied needs for service posed by such persons, where do we start in order to help? The traditional, substance-abuse provider response is that the addiction/dependency is the overall central problem: if we can get the drinking/drugging under control, it will buy the needed time to address other problems (e.g., housing, income, etc.). The hook for attracting and maintaining clients for most of the projects in the cooperative agreement was the provision of housing, food, health care and other services, all of which could be lost if the client did not adhere to the sobriety standard.

For the many homeless who are not amenable to residential interventions (Chicago, this volume), intensive case management may provide the required support and stability that will enable these people eventually to achieve sobriety and employment and thereby to compete for available housing. However, when the problems are long-term, chronic and severe as is the case for many clients in Seattle, the term of treatment in such cases is probably very long (Seattle, this volume).

Huebner and Scott noted further that there is at least one alternative point of view regarding which shall be the primary and which shall be the supportive services for such clients, and this point of view is represented by the Seattle project's model. This model states that while the individual's addiction is an important problem, his (her) homeless status is a more critical and urgent crisis which (1) must be dealt with before any attempt at treating the addiction is made, and (2) must be handled in an "unconditional" manner (i.e., housing and other services continue regardless of the client's drinking or treatment status).

A major barrier to the success of all of these projects is that there is a dearth of permanent housing available to the poor even if the goals of sobriety, employment, and improved mental health have been achieved. To make addiction treatment programs for the homeless most effective, these projects should have a stock of low income housing to which to refer their successful clients. In most of the communities described herein, obtaining such housing is problematic at best. The following sections of this synthesis focus on other theoretical and experiential themes that were covered in the chapters.

POLITICAL ISSUES

One of the important themes running through the chapters is that political issues and turf battles may be major barriers to the initial implementation and the ongoing success of research demonstration projects like those described here. The New Orleans project provides an interesting case study in how the roadblocks of cronyism, racial politics, and turf can be dealt with successfully to establish a working service delivery and research collaboration.

The case of Newark offers an open, insiders' view of how turf battles eventually ground the project to an early halt. On the other hand, in New

Haven a process of coalition building was successful in setting up a viable working partnership that enabled the research and clinical interests to complement each other. For those chapters that expand on the political aspects of their program implementation, one message comes through loud and clear: involve and communicate with all stakeholders in the program and attempt to obtain support at the highest administrative levels. The problems experienced in New Orleans and New Haven appeared to have been mitigated through a process of coalition building where all parties could agree that the project would meet at least some of their goals.

It is also clear that the public needs education on issues of substance abuse treatment. Site selection in several cities involved choosing a location in a neighborhood that "wouldn't notice." In such cases, there is the risk that the neighborhood will not be conducive to the maintenance of sobriety. In other cases a lengthy process of negotiation and public education was needed before the "not in my back yard" (NIMBY) syndrome was overcome (e.g., New Orleans, Tucson). In the Evanston/VA project, national and local VA chiefs of services were involved early on to ensure that they could and would accommodate a new, controversial, residential program on a residential, hospital campus.

SPECIAL POPULATIONS

These projects have resulted in the development of treatment programs for the homeless in some states which had no previous services available for certain populations. In Seattle, public inebriates showed a lack of responsiveness to standard treatments before the funding of this current project began. In St. Louis there were no programs for homeless women with children before this round of demonstration projects.

The St. Louis project has increased the Salvation Army's attention and resources in regard to service delivery to substance abusing mothers and their children. Offering such parenting and childcare services within a substance abuse treatment facility is a fairly new and needed innovation. A significant barrier for many women currently seeking substance abuse treatment is that they must give up their children upon entry into the rehabilitation program. Odyssey House in New York City (Cusky et al., 1979) was one of the first treatment programs to eliminate this barrier. Leipman et al. (1982) have noted that health and family issues appear to offer increased motivational options in working with women that are not present in traditional male-focused programs.

Developing strategies for addressing the recovery needs of women while attending to the needs of their children is an important theoretical development. While many of the present programs are open to women, with notable exceptions they are actually predominantly male.

Some projects allowed women but not children (e.g., Tucson and Albuquerque). Only two projects (Los Angeles and New Orleans) specifically included family interventions in the treatment planning even when children were not in the program. This family treatment is intended to work to heal some of the disruption in family relationships secondary to the substance abuse. The present focus of projects dealing with women and children appears to be on the needs of the women to be parents rather than on needs and outcomes of the affected children. Some outcome studies of the effects of interventions on children are needed. There are many unanswered questions. How old can the children be? What about gender balance? What about educational issues? Are different parenting skills, and teaching methods needed? Are they effective?

As is the case regarding gender or family status, ethnicity can be a major factor in defining patterns of alcohol and drug use and in the corresponding patterns of treatment. For example, the needs, perspectives, and social networks of younger African Americans addicted to crack cocaine will differ from those of older white skid-row-type alcoholics, and neither of these groups will have the same characteristics as chemically dependent Mexican Americans and Native Americans. Albuquerque presents this perspective well and illustrates that projects should develop and maintain cultural sensitivity including a multi-ethnic and multi-lingual staff that represents well the often diverse characteristics of the treatment population.

The co-occurrence of mental illness and substance abuse can also have a major impact on how alcohol and drug treatment services are provided (Christie et al., 1988 and Schukit, 1979). Clients who are homeless and also have these two disorders simultaneously are described as "dually diagnosed" and they represent a subgroup of the homeless population which is especially difficult to treat.

The dually diagnosed homeless may represent as much as one-third of the homeless population (Los Angeles, this volume). This type of individual often "falls through the cracks" and does not receive any services since the two types of disorders are usually treated in separate service systems each with in- and out-patient modalities. The Los Angeles project is concentrating on a dually diagnosed population which is primarily young, white males with schizophrenia or bipolar disorder while the Washington, D.C. project is working primarily with severely mentally ill minority women. The Evanston/VA project, in contrast to Los Angeles and Washington, D.C. whose target populations are 100% dually diagnosed, is working with a target population which is 30% dually diagnosed. The most frequently occurring diagnosis of the Evanston/VA population is major depression. Evanston/VA's target population consists primarily of black male veterans.

Veterans are estimated to represent approximately one-third of homeless men in America. Although several projects have veterans in their sample populations by chance, Evanston/VA is the only demonstration project which deals exclusively with homeless veterans.

OUTREACH

A key to a successful program is the enrollment of the most appropriate target population. Tucson notes that doing this involved meetings with referral agencies on several occasions to familiarize them with the new program, its goals and the criteria defining the target population. Additionally, Tucson hired outreach workers to conduct street outreach to parks, soup kitchens, and so on to make direct contact with needy, hard-to-reach individuals.

As noted earlier, the Seattle project treats chronic public inebriates without recourse to residential care. Seattle acknowledges that the hard-to-treat homeless are often, perhaps usually, not ready for treatment. Therefore, they offer a long term, community-based intervention designed to promote incremental improvement with eventual readiness for sobriety, employment, and housing. Outreach efforts like Seattle's would offer the possibility of ongoing meaningful engagement of hard-to-treat clients which may also be an important component of residential care programs.

In Seattle the case management intervention is individual specific, not group-oriented; focused on assuring client survival and health needs, not on drinking behavior. It emphasizes maintaining a positive connection between the client and the case manager that causes the potential, but not the requirement, for eventual movement towards a drug-free lifestyle. This is a very different set of assumptions from the group-oriented, residential programs in the cooperative agreement. In these projects substance abuse could not be tolerated because it would destroy the imposed order assumed to be a necessary foundation for the recovery of people whose lives were out of control. In the group-oriented programs, empowerment of clients is a gradual process whereby control of one's life is transferred incrementally from the group-enforced system to the increasingly, internally-controlled client.

RELAPSE/RETENTION POLICY

One central consideration on which there is much variation is relapse policy. For example, the New Orleans project appears to accept relapse as a normal part of coping with and managing sobriety. Although the striving for sobriety is required, a relapse is viewed as "grist for the mill," a learning experience. Additionally, Seattle, which treats chronic public inebriates, has no relapse policy since abstinence and sobriety are neither emphasized nor expected. Their main goals are to stabilize their clients and prevent further deterioration. On the other hand are the group-oriented, residential projects where relapse results in termination from the program. There is some variation in the number of relapses necessary for termination with Albuquerque allowing none, and Chicago and Evanston/VA allowing one. Los Angeles's relapse policy relies on individually set goals.

In refining their relapse policies, it appears that the designers of the various residential programs struggled with finding a compromise between the needs of the program environment (drug free) and the recognition that the recovery process for homeless substance abusing individuals is a road fraught with setbacks. Two of the program elements in the Albuquerque project report, in preliminary data, that relapse was the primary reason for discharge. When the needs of the individual predominate, as is the case when only case management is used, a less stringent relapse policy is the most realistic. On the other hand, when the needs of the group predominate, as in residential treatment, a more stringent policy seems to be required. The tougher policy appears to be useful not just to the internal program group but also to outside parties (i.e., neighbors living near the supported residence) in programs that utilize supported independent housing. We should also make the point that, ideally, a continuum of care is available. For example, in the Evanston/VA project, when clients were discharged from or left the residential component, they were still maintained in the case management component for the duration of the one year treatment period.

Philadelphia and Los Angeles make the point that successful program completion is dependent, to some extent, upon readiness to engage in recovery. Program clarification and communication with potential clients at the outset may help to match better the appropriate clients to particular interventions. Los Angeles employed what they believed was a successful strategy for testing potential clients' readiness. They used a two week waiting period between the time of screening and assignment to treatment with the actual beginning of service.

One question regarding this kind of self-selection is whether the more severely impaired and/or hard-to-treat may miss their opportunity for treatment by having to wait for the initiation of service. It will be interesting to observe the people who were initially screened and examine differences between those who were actually admitted to the study versus those who were not.

RESIDENTIAL SERVICES

Many of the demonstration projects emphasized that transitional housing was required to effectively treat homeless persons with substance abuse problems. Since detoxification followed by discharge back into the community where the abuse was occurring is thought to thwart recovery, providing a structured residential experience was proposed to facilitate recovery. Ten projects included a residential component, but there was considerable variation in the type of housing provided. Several projects attempted to provide independent housing (e.g., Chicago, Tucson). Others developed program housing that was similar to independent housing (e.g., New Orleans, Albuquerque) in terms of its location and design. Two projects, however, developed residential housing that was dissimilar to independent housing. The New Haven project uses a 90-day stay in a shelter as its residential component. The Evanston/VA project uses a three to six month stay in a domiciliary-type facility on the grounds of a VA hospital.

Housing appears to be the program component most likely to generate implementation barriers. In Tucson, even door-to-door canvassing was unable to finally sway neighbors to accept the residential program. After narrowly losing a vote, project staff had to utilize housing units already zoned for another project. Similar stories occurred at the other sites. Even the Evanston/VA (VA) site experienced 'NIMBY'-like problems regarding worries about project-clients' presence on the VA Medical Center campus.

One ongoing debate in housing research is between the relative efficacy of transitional and supported housing. Transitional housing is intended as a relatively short-term bridge from homelessness to a more permanent residence. Supported housing on the other hand, is represented as a long term housing intervention in which support services are provided over an extended period of time to help clients remain in a stable residential environment. Most of the present demonstration projects evaluate forms of transitional housing. These residential services range from 90-days to one-year. A number of programs refer clients to supported housing alternatives at discharge from the experimental program. The limits of a three-year collaborative demonstration project do not allow for the study of residential alternatives that are intended to be long-term interventions. Thus the present set of projects may address whether or not transitional housing interventions are effective with persons who are homeless with substance use disorder; however, it will be unable to assess the relative efficacy of residential services intended for durations of more than one year.

CASE MANAGEMENT

Case management has been utilized in both rounds of cooperative demonstration programs funded by NIAAA (Huebner et al., this volume). In the first round of research demonstrations, funded in 1987, four of nine projects utilized case management; and of the four which utilized case management, two projects tested the effectiveness of case management using experimental designs (Willenbring et al., 1991). In the second round of demonstration projects, funded by NIAAA in 1990, all 14 projects included some form of case management in their program design.

The various case management models developed by the 14 projects all share similar functions; however, they differ on how these functions are performed. The component functions of case management include outreach, assessment, treatment planning, linkage, monitoring and evaluation, client advocacy, crisis intervention, resource development, the provision of aftercare services, client advocacy, service brokering (system advocacy), supportive counseling, practical support, and program linkage. How these functions are performed can be characterized along various continuous dimensions going from one pole to another (see Willenbring et al., 1991). For example, the intensity of the case management intervention is a dimension that refers to the frequency of contact and the ratio of staff to clients. In the Cooperative Agreement Program there are several projects which describe their interventions as utilizing "intensive case management." Generally, sites used this adjective if the client/staff ratio was 20:1 or less. The lowest such ratio occurred at the Denver site where two case managers shared 17 clients. As an example of a more typical situation, the highest client/staff ratio occurred at the Philadelphia site control group where 70 control clients were assigned to one case manager.

Other dimensions which vary in the case management interventions include the site of service, the amount of training of the case managers and the case management team structure. The Seattle project delivers case management services in the field while the Philadelphia and St. Louis projects (among others) deliver case manager services at shelters. Other projects such as Evanston/VA and Denver have their own free standing facilities where both residential and case management services are provided simultaneously. Case management training varies from advanced professional degrees (Evanston/VA) to on the job training (St. Louis). Team structure also varies from that where a primary case manager has their own caseload (Seattle, Evanston/VA) to a team model where case managers share clients (Denver has dyads or pairs of case managers which share 17 clients).

In contrast to the area of mental health, research on case management in alcohol and drug treatment has only tentatively demonstrated effectiveness or explored what functions might account for it (Willenbring et al., 1991). Therefore, results from the ongoing and final evaluations of the Cooperative Agreement Program will be extremely helpful to clinicians and policy makers involved in this aspect of public health.

TRANSITION TO INDEPENDENCE

Policymakers should take note of the Birmingham project's enhanced day treatment program which has both work and housing components. This project seems to offer a relatively inexpensive and effective way of rehabilitating low cost housing which is then offered to homeless clients who have remained drug and alcohol free for a certain length of time. Such a program could be duplicated elsewhere if such low cost housing were available.

IMPLICATIONS FOR RESEARCH

Several of the projects discussed the fact that the random assignment of subjects to experimental and control conditions was problematic for project staff, clients, and researchers. This issue is not trivial, but deserves careful attention in future studies of community-based interventions. These types of problems with the research design may actually reduce the interpretability of the experimental findings. While space does not permit a detailed discussion of this issue here, we thought it was important to mention its existence, and that we, and other participants in the Cooperative Agreement Program intend to discuss it further in subsequent papers.

However, a strength of the Cooperative Agreement Program was that data collection did not rely on the randomized experimental design alone. Rather, in addition to longitudinal outcome measures, detailed quantitative and qualitative utilization and process data were collected to enable more complex studies of the relationships among client characteristics, service utilization, program characteristics, and client outcomes.

Process evaluation for program improvement. Several sites (Philadelphia, Evanston/VA, and Washington, D.C.) stressed the importance of including process evaluation as an integral part of program implementation. Research and program staff should work together early on to choose appropriate *qualitative and quantitative* variables to be measured during the course of the project. Timely feedback to the clinical program from both staff and clients can improve the effectiveness of the program. For example, the Evanston/VA project used process data to study the effects of a revision of the pass policy which seemed to be effective in lowering the relapse rate.

Process data are valuable in continuous quality improvement efforts and in informing training of staff. Continuous in-service training for staff involved in chemical dependency is extremely important in maintaining the intervention as it was planned as well as preventing staff burnout. The St. Louis project found it advantageous to educate all staff including janitors and clerical help. This adjustment was made after clients of the St. Louis project pointed out that they could "outwit staff."

Regarding future demonstration projects of this type, one recommendation would be to increase the length of such projects from three to five years. Three years is probably too short a time to adequately implement and evaluate interventions or treatment programs which are meant to change human behavior when it involves long term chemical dependency often compounded by mental illness. For example, it may take one to two years for a case management team to mature and stabilize.

THE COOPERATIVE AGREEMENT

This NIAAA Cooperative Agreement Program has had many unusual, noteworthy and constructive characteristics that deserve mention here. First of all, it mandated that rigorous research be integral to the projects with a researcher as principal investigator (P.I.). While several of the authors have noted problems with the implementation of the research designs that were used, we view these as important lessons to be learned from and improved upon. While the design and implementation of rigorous research in studies of human services needs improvement, the principle of careful, systematic, well planned data collection and analysis was employed in exemplary fashion in this Cooperative Agreement Program. Rigorous quantitative and qualitative scientific methods such as those employed in the Cooperative Agreement Program are essential to improving the theory and implementation of social programs.

While researchers served as P.I.'s, the clinical project directors were treated as co-equal Co-P.I.'s. This facilitated cooperation between research and clinical components of the research demonstrations. The fostering of communication and cooperation was a key to the high success rate in the implementation and continuation of these projects.

The national evaluation staff from NIAAA, R.O.W. Sciences, and the Vanderbilt Institute for Public Policy Studies was active in facilitating and monitoring the implementation of both research and clinical components through yearly site visits and semi-annual working group meetings of all sites in Washington, D.C. The national working group meetings were very useful in communicating among projects about problems and progress and in learning from each other. This book is a direct result of these meetings, and we expect that more collaborative products will result from the cooperation and communication that has developed directly from these national working group meetings.

In conclusion, we were very pleased to represent the fine group of researchers and practitioners that participated in the Cooperative Agreement Program. We enjoyed the process and learned an immense amount from our participation. We hope that this book enables readers to share some of the benefits of this rich experience.

REFERENCES

Christie, K., Burke, J., Regier, D., Rea, D., Boyd, J., and Locke, B. (1988). Epidemiologic Evidence for the Early Onset of Mental Disorders and Higher Risk of Drug Abuse In Young Adults. *Am. J. Psychiatry.* 145: 971-975.

Cusky, W. R., Richardson, A. H., & Berger, L. H. (1979). *Specialized therapeutic community program for female addicts,* D.H.H.S. Pub No. (ADM 79-880, Government Printing Office), Washington, D.C.

Leipman, M. R., Wolper, B., Vazquez, J. (1982). An ecological approach for motivating women to accept treatment for drug dependency. *Treatment services for drug dependent women,* National Institute of Drug Abuse, Government Printing Office, Washington, D.C.

Schukit, M. A. (1979). *Drug and Alcohol Abuse.* New York: Plenum.

Willenbring, M. L., Ridgely, M. S., Stinchfield, R. and Rose, B.A. (1991). *Application of Case Management in Alcohol and Drug Dependence: Matching Techniques and Populations.* Prepared for the U.S. Department of H.H.S., Rockville, MD, Contract #89MF00933901D.

Index